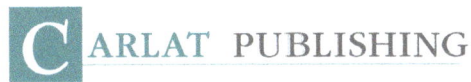

Psychiatry Practice Boosters, Fourth Edition

Edited by Jesse Koskey, MD
Associate Editor: Zachary Davis

Published by Carlat Publishing, LLC
PO Box 626, Newburyport, MA 01950

Copyright © 2023 All Rights Reserved.

Publisher and Editor-in-Chief: Daniel Carlat, MD
Deputy Editor: Talia Puzantian, PharmD, BCPP
Senior Editor: Ilana Fogelson
Associate Editor: Harmony Zambrano

All rights reserved. This book is protected by copyright.

This CME/CE activity is intended for psychiatrists, psychiatric nurses, psychologists, and other health care professionals with an interest in mental health. The Carlat CME Institute is accredited by the Accreditation Council for Continuing Medical Education to provide continuing medical education for physicians. Carlat CME Institute maintains responsibility for this program and its content. The American Board of Psychiatry and Neurology has reviewed *Psychiatry Practice Boosters* and has approved this program as a comprehensive Self-Assessment and CME Program, which is mandated by ABMS as a necessary component of maintenance of certification. Carlat CME Institute designates this enduring material educational activity for a maximum of four (4) ABPN Maintenance of Certification credits as part of the 2024 course. Physicians or psychologists should claim credit commensurate only with the extent of their participation in the activity. CME quizzes must be taken online at www.thecarlatreport.com.

Carlat Publishing books are available at special quantity discounts for bulk purchases as premiums, for fund-raising, or for educational use. To order, visit www.thecarlatreport.com or call 866-348-9279.

Print ISBN: *979-8-9873354-6-8*
eBook ISBN: *979-8-9873354-5-1*

2 3 4 5 6 7 8 9 10

Table of Contents

Acknowledgments vi
Introduction vii
A Quick Primer on Assessing Scientific Research 1

ADDICTION PSYCHIATRY 7
- Antipsychotics for Methamphetamine Psychosis 8
- Buprenorphine Induction Without Withdrawal 10
- Gabapentin for Alcohol Use Disorder, Redux 12
- Internet-Based Approaches for Gambling Problems 14
- Is AA the Toast of the Town? 16
- Meds for Alcohol Use Disorder 18
- A Novel Treatment for Methamphetamine Use Disorder 20
- Opioid Agonist Treatment and Decreased Mortality 22
- Should Prolonged Abstinence From Alcohol Be Required Before Liver Transplant? 24
- Smoking Cessation Intervention for Hospitalized Patients 26
- Starting Buprenorphine: Is Timing Everything? 28
- Stigmatizing Smoking: An Effective Deterrent? 29
- Sublocade vs SL Buprenorphine After Release From Jail 30
- Suboxone vs Vivitrol for Opioid Use Disorder 32

CHILD AND ADOLESCENT PSYCHIATRY 35
- ADHD Prevalence in Black American Children 36
- Can Stimulants Prevent Crime? 37
- Clozapine for Conduct Disorder in Schizophrenia 38
- DASH Diet for Childhood ADHD 39
- The Effect of Age and Pubertal Stage on Mental Health in Gender-Incongruent Youth 41
- Electroconvulsive Therapy in Adolescents and Transitional-Age Youth 43
- The Evidence for Polypharmacy in ADHD 45
- Intravenous Ketamine for Teen Depression 47
- Long-Term Treatment Response in Pediatric OCD 48

- New Canadian Guidelines for Eating Disorders in Children 50
- A Novel Treatment for Dramatic-Onset Autoimmune OCD or Severe Food Restriction? . . . 51
- SSRIs and Hydroxyzine for Avoidant/Restrictive Food Intake Disorder? 53
- Viloxazine for ADHD in Children and Adolescents 55
- Vitamin D for ADHD? 57
- Which Medications Have the Lowest Risk of Side Effects? 59

GERIATRIC PSYCHIATRY 61
- Does Mirtazapine Treat Agitation in Dementia? 62
- Less Sleep Correlated With Dementia 64
- Listening to Depression: The Importance of Addressing Hearing Loss 65
- Low Vitamin B_{12} Associated With Depression in Older Adults 66
- Rest Easy: Benzos, Z-Drugs, and Dementia 67
- SSRIs and Intracerebral Hemorrhage Risk 69

MANAGING ADVERSE EFFECTS 71
- Anticholinergic-Associated Cognitive Impairment in Schizophrenia 72
- Antidepressants Harm Some With Bipolar Depression 74
- Antipsychotic Dosing: How High? 76
- Antipsychotic Use Associated With Increased Risk of Mortality 78
- Beta-Blockers and Depression: The Controversy Revisited 80
- Comparison of GI Side Effects of Antidepressants 82
- Do Structural Brain Abnormalities Predict Cognitive Impairment With Electroconvulsive Therapy? 84
- Lithium Exposure In Utero: How Bad Is It Really? 86
- New Combination Treatment Mitigates Antipsychotic-Induced Weight Gain 88
- Omega-3s and Metabolic Risks in Schizophrenia 90
- Polypharmacy in Schizophrenia 92
- A Single Prescriber Reduces Risk of Overdose in Patients on Opioids and Benzodiazepines 94
- Vitamin B_6 Lowers Prolactin on Antipsychotics 95

MOOD DISORDERS 97
- An Answer for Psychotic Depression 98

- Antidepressants for Suicidal Ideation in Depressed Patients?...................99
- Aripiprazole in Depression: The Right Dose............................100
- Brexpiprazole Does Not Treat Mania...................................101
- Can Antidepressants Prolong Survival in Cancer Patients?.................103
- Can We Treat Depression by Targeting Inflammation?....................105
- How Essential Is Antidepressant Continuation?..........................106
- Lumateperone in Bipolar Depression...................................108
- Optimal Antidepressant Doses in Major Depression......................110
- Oral Zuranolone for Postpartum Depression............................112
- Quetiapine in Bipolar With OCD.....................................114
- Psilocybin: The New Holy Grail for the Rapid Relief of Major Depression?......115
- The Role of rTMS in Post-Stroke Depression...........................117

PTSD 119
- Shining a Light on PTSD...120
- Two Negative Studies of Mirtazapine and Riluzole for PTSD in Veterans........122

About Carlat Publishing 124

Acknowledgments

It was a privilege to edit this edition of *Practice Boosters*. And it was a task to consider which of the hundreds of research updates from the past three years of Carlat and its permutations (addictions, child, geriatric, and hospital) were the most interesting, practice-changing, and relevant. The final selections run the gamut from the FDA's newest psychiatric medication approvals to some disappointing (but informative) negative trials, crossing an array of subspecialties and practice settings. I hope that breadth, and the down-to-earth, concise overviews, combine to make for high-yield reading.

I am grateful to our fantastic team at Carlat Publishing, especially the invaluable assistance of Zachary Davis. This project also could not have happened without support from my wife Kee.

The original research updates adapted for this publication were authored by:

Chris Aiken, MD	James Jenkins, MD	Michael Posternak, MD
Deepti Anbarasan, MD	Thomas Jordan, MD	John C. Raiss, MD
Rehan Aziz, MD	Gregory Lande, MD	Sean Ransom, PhD
Sonya Bakshi, MD	Anne Li, MD	Nicholas Rosenlicht, MD
Paul Barkopoulos, MD	Jesus Ligot, MD	Talya Shahal, MD
James Black, MD	Pavan Madan, MD	Susan Siegfreid, MD
Peter J. Farago, MD	C. Jason Mallo, DO	Batya Swift Yasgur, MA, LSW
Kamron Fariba, MD	Brian Miller, MD, PhD, MPH	Lara Tang, MD
Joshua Feder, MD	Richard Moldawski, MD	Amy Ton, MD
Kristen Gardner, PharmD	David Moltz, MD	Sanya Virani, MD
Heather Goff, MD	Randall Moore, MD	Dax Volle, MD
Christina Guest, MD	Susie Morris, MD	Mikveh Warshaw, NP
Victoria Hendrick, MD	Benjamin Oldfield, MD	
Edmund Higgins, MD	John O'Neal, MD	

Introduction

Do you sometimes wish you were a pathologist? Or an oncologist? Imagine *seeing* what ails your patients on a cellular level—visualizing the pathophysiology of depression or psychosis. Or knowing *exactly* how a drug targets and ameliorates the processes that cause symptoms. Or being sure of which side effects patients will experience and how long treatment will take.

Clinical psychiatry can seem pretty primitive at times. That may be part of the appeal. Every patient and treatment course is unique because there is so much variety in the genes, environments, and brains of our patients. This requires us to consider both the stories our patients tell *and* the best evidence we have for a particular diagnosis. Sometimes this means relying on the knowledge base we've been using for years. Sometimes this means expanding that knowledge base, or rejecting it.

That's hard to do when you're working full time with patients, or teaching, or researching—not to mention "just" balancing work and life.

That's where we hope this book can be most helpful. *The Carlat Psychiatry Report* and the *Addiction Treatment, Child Psychiatry, Geriatric Psychiatry,* and *Hospital Psychiatry* reports are pithy, clinically focused psychiatric news digests. Research updates (RUs) are a staple of each issue: careful examinations of new studies with real-world implications. For this book, we collected the most relevant, impactful, and significant RUs from all five Carlat reports over the last few years. We weighed them from a clinical perspective and, when possible, updated them with the most recent data. We feel this collection is the best of the best of Carlat—a boiled-down extract of essential evidence to keep you up to date, engaged, and enjoying your practice as a psychiatrist, psychologist, psychiatric NP, PA, or other mental health professional.

For each RU, we give you a summary of the background, methods, findings, and significance. We address any quality-related or methodological limitations. And we end with the "Carlat take" and "Practice implications," giving you a quick takeaway of both the study and its relevance to practice.

For this edition of *Practice Boosters*, we've also revised our primer on scientific research to include more study designs while doing our best to stay as concise as possible.

We hope that you'll agree with our analyses and recommendations, whether or not they change your practice. That will always come down to your clinical judgment regarding the patient in front of you. But generally speaking, we suggest that if a clinical trial is very large and shows a marked advantage of a new treatment over placebo (or another first-line treatment), it should probably find its way into your toolbox. If a study is small, we recommend it if there aren't significant risks or many other options. If the study has practice-changing potential, but is small or otherwise problematic, we want you to know about it, but we usually recommend a wait-and-see approach.

A Quick Primer on Assessing Scientific Research

THERE'S A REASON you (probably) don't take the latest issue of *JAMA Psychiatry* or *PLOS ONE* to the beach. Scientific research is rarely written with an ear for language, let alone entertainment. It has its own jargon, and statistics can be a language unto itself. This book is intended to help you translate the research and get to the bottom of what's relevant in psychiatry. But most clinicians will at some point take their own look at the papers most relevant to their work. This takes practice, and it can help to have a method. To that end, here's a systematic approach to reading and evaluating scientific studies, adapted from "How to Read a Journal Article" by Dr. Jeffrey Barkin, originally published in the February 2007 *Carlat Psychiatry Report*.

ACCESSING SCIENTIFIC PAPERS

All of the articles referenced in this book can be located by entering the title into the search bar at PubMed (www.pubmed.ncbi.nlm.nih.gov). Some of these studies are available to anyone. For others, PubMed will provide an abstract, but the full article will require a one-time purchase, journal subscription, or institutional access. You may also find that their authors welcome correspondence and are willing to share their research with you via email.

GENERAL TIPS

There's no need to read each word of a study sequentially, as one does for fiction. Jumping around and revisiting sentences and sections is helpful. And just like for children's books, you may want to spend a while with the pictures and their captions. The core argument of the paper is often laid out in charts and figures. Research papers *are* arguments; their authors are marshaling—sometimes to a fault—the data and interpretations that they feel are necessary to convince readers that a hypothesis has either been proven or refuted. Read studies skeptically, therefore, as if you are preparing to debate the study authors. There are career-related and financial incentives for authors to publish, not just altruistic ones. Even if that weren't the case, cognitive biases can skew data in ways we don't recognize until after the fact. Here are some rubrics by which you should evaluate scientific papers:

1. Who funded the study?

If a study is funded by a drug manufacturer, it is more likely to report results favorable to the sponsor's drug (Lundh A et al, *Cochrane Database Syst Rev* 2012;12:MR000033). The reasons for this are not necessarily nefarious. Industry-funded studies are often very well designed, with large numbers of subjects and gold-standard research methods. One reason companies are more likely to get positive results is that they are careful about which drugs they choose to study. Often they will start with a very small feasibility study before deciding that a particular compound is worth the financial outlay for a large randomized trial. Company-paid scientists do sometimes engage in research trickery, such as setting up a control group for failure by providing a low dose of a comparison drug, or changing their statistical analyses after the fact.

Bottom line: While industry-funded studies can be valuable, give their conclusions more scrutiny than those funded by more objective sources, such as the National Institute of Mental Health or private foundations.

2. What is being studied?

In other words, what are the identified primary and secondary outcomes of the study? Good randomized controlled trials (RCTs) test a hypothesis by identifying, in advance of data gathering, the single primary outcome that the researchers will focus on. Often researchers will identify secondary outcomes as well. Declaring all these outcomes in advance, along with study methods, is the best-case scenario: It keeps researchers from trying to "hack" data by doing post-hoc analyses and crunching numbers until they stumble across a formula that produces a "significant" result that actually happened by chance. *Not all significant results accurately convey what happened in the study or answer the initial hypothesis.*

Imagine an RCT of drug X versus placebo for adults with major depressive disorder (MDD). Researchers decide in advance that their primary outcome will be Patient Health Questionnaire (PHQ-9) scores after two months of treatment for their two groups, and their secondary outcome will be subjective self-reports of hours slept. They enroll a study population of adults who have MDD but don't have bipolar disorder, psychotic disorders, etc. (the usual exclusion criteria) and conduct their study.

If the researchers find that there was no difference in PHQ-9 scores between the two groups, they must conclude that drug X is not an effective antidepressant. This is not necessarily bad news—it helps us know more about drug X. However, the researchers might have been hoping to publish something that changes how depression is treated. If they find that drug X improved patient self-reported sleep versus placebo, that is interesting too. They might title their study and write their report around the finding that for adults with depression, drug X is associated with improved sleep. Depending on the context, that might be information that influences clinical practice. (To really hang our hats on drug X for sleep in MDD, though, we'd prefer a study designed around that as a primary outcome, not a secondary one.)

Now imagine that the researchers continue to analyze their data beyond those primary and secondary outcomes. If they find that for women between ages 20 and 30, drug X was associated with an improvement in appetite, how helpful is that? We're getting pretty hypothetical here, and the real answer would rely on the actual data, but generally speaking, it's likely to just be a statistical fluke. One would want an RCT of women ages 20–30 taking drug X vs placebo and reporting a primary outcome of appetite to know that the outcome is "real" and reflects what actually happened to the study participants.

Bottom line: Focus on the results of predefined primary outcomes when interpreting results from trials.

3. Who is being studied?

Many trials have strict inclusion and exclusion criteria. Their results may, therefore, not apply to the patients in your office. For example, antidepressant trials often exclude patients with symptoms that are too mild or too severe, or patients with comorbid substance use, bipolar disorder, psychosis, or suicidality. Additionally, systemic bias excludes many patient populations from psychiatric research. One study concluded that patients who make it into research trials represent only about 20% of the patients whom real clinicians actually treat (Zimmerman M et al, *Am J Psychiatry* 2005;162(7):1370–1372). For smaller studies, or those that challenge accepted practice, give more consideration to the relevance for a given patient in your office.

Pay attention to how the researchers deal with patients who drop out of a study. This happens for various reasons, such as adverse events or clinical worsening, and there are different ways to account for it. The most conservative is called **last observation carried forward** (LOCF). In RCTs, LOCF is also called **intention-to-treat** (ITT) analysis. In these methods, each subject's last score is included, regardless of when the subject dropped out. If an antidepressant causes early dropouts, the LOCF method will drag the depression score down, making the medication appear less effective. This is precisely the kind of information we need to know as clinicians, because the ideal medication should be both efficacious and well tolerated.

By contrast, a less conservative method is **observed cases**, aka "per protocol" analysis. Here, only the subjects who stay in a study until the very end are counted, ignoring all dropouts.

Bottom line: Look for studies that include subjects relevant to your patient, and for LOCF when those participants don't complete the study.

4. How is this hypothesis being tested?

In other words, what's the study design? The most reliable evidence comes from collecting the results of multiple studies (ideally, RCTs) in a **meta-analysis**. These analyses aggregate and analyze the results of studies to assess for trends. Quality meta-analyses will explain how they assess for the presence of bias within individual studies. For example, they will look for evidence of a publication bias, wherein certain findings aren't being publicized. "Garbage in, garbage out" is a good phrase to keep in mind when you consider how reliable a meta-analysis is. The PRISMA (Preferred Reporting Items for Systematic Reviews and Meta-Analyses) guidelines, available online, are an evidence-based rubric for evaluating meta-analyses.

Systematic reviews and **literature reviews** also combine data from multiple studies, but do not necessarily perform statistical analyses. "Garbage in, garbage out" applies to them as well, but reviews can be high-quality guides curated to provide expertise and depth.

So, then, what are these **RCTs** that make up good meta-analyses and reviews? Study populations in RCTs are randomized to different groups (or "arms"), each of which receives a separate intervention. At least one of these arms is a "control," or intervention for which the outcome is already familiar or expected. This can be a placebo or an accepted standard of care.

Randomization allows researchers to minimize the influences of normally occurring variations on an outcome. If you're studying the antidepressant effects of a medication known to have a disparate effect across sexes (by worsening menstrual cramps, for example), you'll only be able to dismiss any between-group effects of that variable if you've got a statistically equal number of men and women in each group. RCTs worth their salt will provide a table that shows the randomization results and relevant characteristics of the people in each study arm.

The control part of RCTs is important, too. It's hard to know how well an intervention works if you don't have anything to compare it with. If you give a toddler a lollipop, and she's happy, maybe that's due to the lollipop. Or maybe it's because she just had a nap. But if you take two toddlers, wake both up after a refreshing nap, and only give a lollipop to one, then you're surer that any reaction is due to the lollipop. (Be a nice researcher—use a crossover design so the other one gets a lollipop too.)

A placebo control is the best way to evaluate the effects of a novel medication. Swallowing a pill on its own has a placebo effect, and researchers control for that effect by giving pills to both groups that are identical in every way except that one contains the medication and the other an inert substance. Now things are as equal as can be. A well-run trial might have groups A and B, both randomized, and group A gets new drug X while group B gets a placebo. With this setup, we know that if A improves more than B in a statistically significant way (more on that below), it's very likely *because of* the presence of drug X.

Blinding further shores up RCT results. In single-blinded studies, the patients do not know whether they got the placebo or the medication. In double-blinded studies, both the patient and the researchers are unaware. Researcher expectations are known to skew outcomes, so double-blinding is the gold standard.

An active drug can also be used as a control, such as when a new antidepressant is tested against a tried-and-true medication like fluoxetine. This sounds like a good idea, but it is a step below placebo control. The problem is that if both groups improve to a similar degree, we don't know if it was all due to the placebo effect. Remember, the placebo is a real treatment. Patients get better in the hands of a well-organized, empathic research team, so much so that the effects of an active medication may be undetectable. For the same reason, it is very hard to show that antidepressants bring any meaningful benefits when added to psychotherapy.

Uncontrolled studies have neither a placebo nor an active drug control. Generally, uncontrolled studies yield response rates that are much higher than those in controlled studies. So why are so many published? Well, much of the research out there is not meant to inform practice—it's meant to inspire new research, hopefully with better designs. There are several types of uncontrolled or "observational" studies, and I'll walk through them from the most reliable designs to the least.

A **cohort study** is a way of doing a controlled trial when it is not possible to randomize patients to groups, for ethical or logistical reasons, or when the intervention or outcome in question has already happened, like a traumatic earthquake. Studies that comb through population health registries or electronic medical records are often cohort studies. These studies usually compare two groups: one that received an exposure or had an outcome of interest, and another that didn't. The relevant data can be gathered prospectively, by following the groups forward, or retrospectively, by looking backward in time.

A typical example of a **prospective cohort study** involves medications in pregnancy. Say researchers identify two groups of depressed women: those who take SSRIs during pregnancy, and those who don't. Then they follow the groups to check for problems. Since it would be unethical to randomize the women, the two groups may differ in significant ways. For example, women who opt to receive SSRIs may be more depressed, or those who opt to not take them may rely more on exercise to treat depression. If this study finds that infants have more neonatal problems after being exposed to SSRIs in the womb, that would be helpful—but the researchers wouldn't be able to know if the problems were caused by the medications, or the severity of depression, or less exercise. That's the main weakness of observational studies when compared with RCTs and the phenomenon behind the popular truism that correlation doesn't mean causation.

If the researchers in this example instead start with children exposed and not exposed to SSRIs in utero, and then assess for the presence of a condition suspected to be related to SSRIs in pregnancy, that would be a **retrospective cohort study**, as it looks backward to the exposure to create the two groups. And if the researchers start with children who have and don't have the condition suspected to be related to SSRIs in pregnancy, and then look backward to see which had been exposed to SSRIs in utero, that would be a **case-control** observational study, as the cases with the condition are compared to the controls without it. As with prospective cohort studies, each of these observational study types has limitations when compared with RCTs.

A **cross-sectional study** is an observational study that looks at data at a single point in time. Researchers might use this method with a large population registry or an electronic medical record to assess the prevalence of a given disease in a given population, or the use of a particular medication.

A **case series** is simply a description of a group of patients—for example, those with a particular illness who have received a particular treatment. This is often retrospective data mined from electronic medical records or registries. These reports are suggestive, but not definitive; nothing causative can be concluded from them.

Case reports are the lowest on the hierarchy. They are reports by doctors of single unusual cases, published in hopes that they'll be helpful either in generating hypotheses or for other clinicians who are treating similar patients. While they're not scientifically robust, they may be informative when there are no better data available.

Bottom line: Start your literature search with high-quality meta-analyses and RCTs and give these the most weight. You can select them as filters when searching PubMed.

5. Are the results statistically *and* clinically significant?

In casual conversation, "significant" means big, but in research it means that the results are likely to be true, even if the results are very small. The larger (or more "powered") the study, the more likely it is that the differences it measures are real. The most common assessment of statistical significance is the **p value**, and the most commonly accepted p value for significance is <0.05, which means it is less than 5% likely that the result in question occurred by chance alone. (A p value of 0.01 means that a chance outcome is 1% likely, 0.2 means 20% likely, etc.) A report will often say something like, "Drug X was significantly better than placebo at improving PHQ-9 scores at two months, with patients in the intervention arm reporting scores that were on average 30% lower (p=0.01)."

Confidence interval (CI) is a related measure of significance. Its threshold is usually set at 95% (like p value) and reported with bracketed lower and upper limits. For example, "Drug X was associated with improved PHQ-9 scores at two months, with patients reporting an average score of 10 points, 95% CI

[9, 13]." In essence, this can be taken to indicate a 95% probability that the true value (as opposed to the calculated one) falls between nine and 13. In this case, since 10 is in that range, the result is significant. If the calculated result had been 15, it would fall outside the range of the 95% CI and therefore not be significant. Just as with p values, a more highly powered study allows for more precise CIs.

Significance is not synonymous with relevance, however. When a study reports that one medication has a "significantly" lower rate of nausea than others, look beyond the p value. If the study is large enough, the p could be <0.0001, but the absolute difference in rates of nausea between drugs could be 5%. How likely is that to change your prescribing?

The **effect size** helps convey how powerful a result is in practice. This is the magnitude of a statistically significant difference. An effect size of zero implies that the result for a treatment group was the same as for a comparison group, ie, that there was no effect at all. Other effect sizes break down as follows:

- 0.0–0.2: little to no effect (eg, vortioxetine in generalized anxiety disorder [GAD])
- 0.2–0.5: small effect (eg, SSRIs in GAD)
- 0.5–0.8: moderate effect (eg, benzodiazepines in GAD)
- ≥0.9: large effect (eg, stimulants in ADHD; electroconvulsive therapy or ketamine in depression)

Effect sizes for psychiatric treatments range from barely detectable (medications for GAD are 0.3; PTSD medications are 0.2) to loud and clear (stimulants in ADHD are 0.7–0.8; exposure therapy for phobias is 1.0). Across all psychiatric treatments, from psychotherapy to medications, the average effect size weighs in at 0.5.

Finally, among all the data and statistics in a paper, look for the **number needed to treat (NNT)** and the **number needed to harm (NNH)**. Like effect sizes, these help tell how clinically applicable a finding is likely to be. NNT is a measurement of how many patients would need to receive an intervention in order for it to be helpful to one of them. NNH is the number of patients treated before one is harmed in a specific way, such as weight gain or dropping out of the study. An NNT of 1 would be ideal, but in practice we generally look for NNTs that are low single digits. However, you might consider higher NNTs for patients with rare or refractory conditions.

Bottom line: Statistical significance is a necessary but not often sufficient condition. Look for absolute differences, effect sizes, and NNTs to gain a more complete understanding of results.

BIBLIOGRAPHY

Gehlbach SH. *Interpreting the Medical Literature*. 5th ed. New York, NY: McGraw-Hill Education / Medical; 2006.

Ghaemi SN. *A Clinician's Guide to Statistics and Epidemiology in Mental Health*. New York, NY: Cambridge University Press; 2009.

Greenhalgh T. *How to Read a Paper: The Basics of Evidence-Based Medicine*. United Kingdom: Wiley; 2014.

ADDICTION PSYCHIATRY

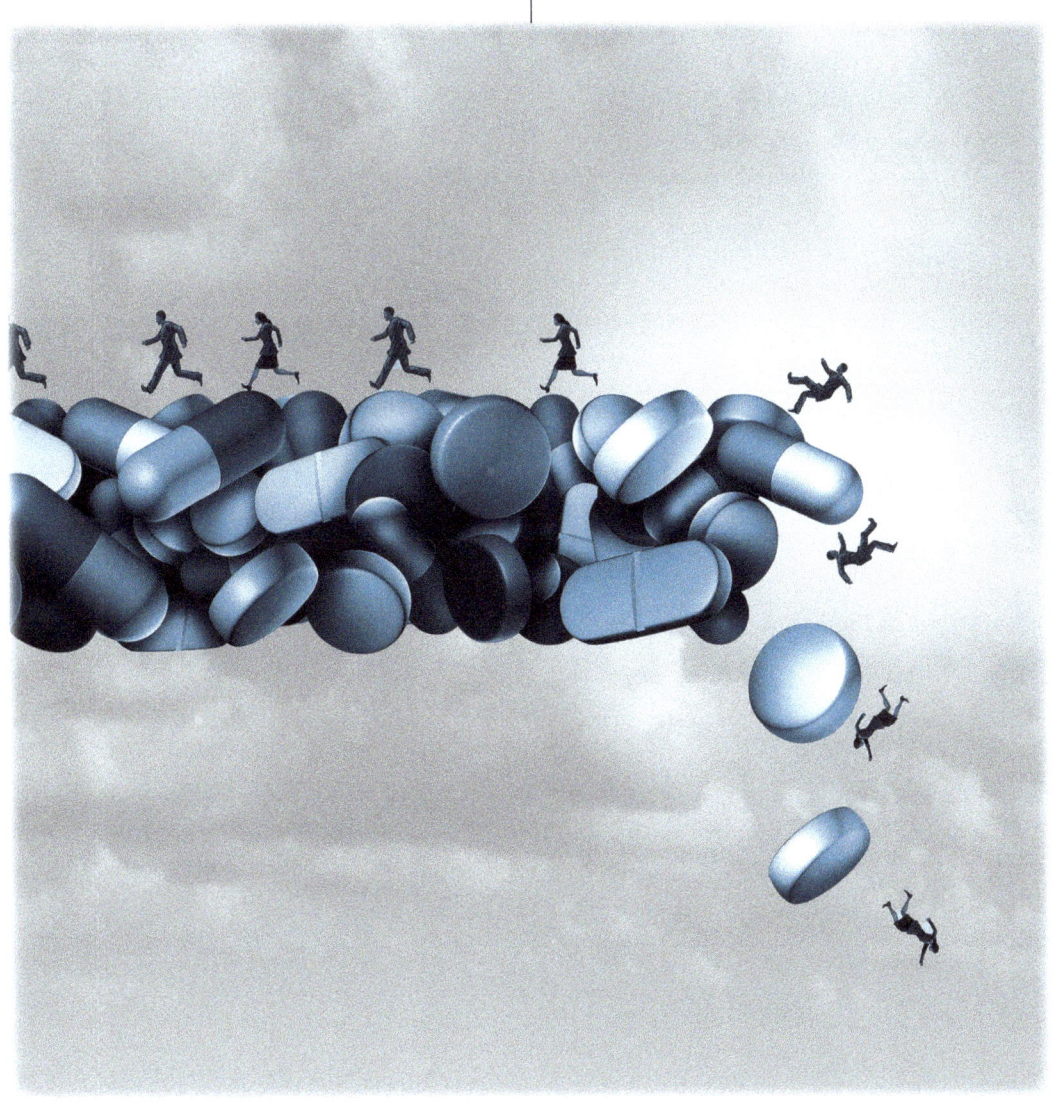

Antipsychotics for Methamphetamine Psychosis

REVIEW OF: Srisurapanont M, Likhitsathian S, Suttajit S, et al. Efficacy and dropout rates of antipsychotic medications for methamphetamine psychosis: A systematic review and network meta-analysis. *Drug Alcohol Depend.* 2021;219:108467.

STUDY TYPE: Systematic review and network meta-analysis

Methamphetamine psychosis (MAP) is difficult to treat. There are only so many antipsychotics in our repertoire, and of the few randomized clinical trials (RCTs) we have of MAP management, no antipsychotic has shown itself to be definitively better than any other. So, what is a clinician to do?

The authors conducted a network meta-analysis of six head-to-head RCTs of antipsychotics for MAP (n=395), in effect creating head-to-head comparisons. The medications were risperidone (four trials, n=129); haloperidol (three trials, n=93); aripiprazole (two trials, n=48); and paliperidone extended release (ER), quetiapine, and olanzapine (one trial each for a total n=125).

The evidence in each trial was judged to be of low or very low quality, and none of the trials individually found significant differences between medications. However, when data from all the trials were pooled, the authors were able to establish somewhat of a hierarchy among them. Comparisons between medications were reported as standardized mean difference (SMD), which is a way of standardizing outcomes across studies that measure similar outcomes in various ways.

RESULTS:

Of all the possible head-to-head medication comparisons, a few significant differences were found. Quetiapine (300 mg/day) and olanzapine (20 mg/day) were superior to risperidone (4–8 mg/day) and aripiprazole (15 mg/day) for psychotic symptoms. Aripiprazole was the big loser—it was inferior to haloperidol (6–20 mg/day) and paliperidone ER (9 mg/day), as well as to quetiapine and olanzapine.

The authors acknowledged that only six RCTs met their inclusion criteria, and the total n did not allow for robust conclusions to be drawn from all drug comparisons. Other shortcomings included the lack of placebo control and overall study heterogeneity.

The authors pointed out that the D2 receptor blockade caused by these medications in the setting of methamphetamine withdrawal could heighten anhedonia and at least theoretically increase risk of return to drug use. Hyperphagia and hypersomnia resulting from methamphetamine withdrawal might compound the side effects from olanzapine and quetiapine. Given that MAP is often self-limiting, the recommendation is to taper off the antipsychotic after resolution of psychotic symptoms, typically a maximum of four weeks after methamphetamine use.

CARLAT TAKE:

This study attempted an end run around the "garbage in, garbage out" rule of thumb for meta-analyses. Given the low quality of available evidence, it at least gives us a place to start when treating MAP.

PRACTICE IMPLICATIONS:

Consider quetiapine and olanzapine first when treating patients for MAP. Consider tapering when patients are symptom-free and four weeks out from their last methamphetamine use.

Buprenorphine Induction Without Withdrawal

REVIEW OF: Ahmed S, Bhivandkar S, Lonergan BB, Suzuki J. Microinduction of buprenorphine/naloxone: A review of the literature. *Am J Addict.* 2021;30(4):305–315.

STUDY TYPE: Literature review

Buprenorphine is notorious for precipitating withdrawal in patients who have recently taken opioids. Its high receptor affinity and partial agonism at the mu receptor can make inductions tricky: Giving it too soon can cause severe withdrawal; giving it too late means patients have been in discomfort from withdrawal while awaiting their first buprenorphine dose. A fair number of inductions result in some level of precipitated withdrawal (estimates range from 5% to 16.8%), and it has been speculated that higher prevalence of fentanyl on the street has increased this rate even further. But there may be an alternative.

This review examined a novel approach called "microinduction" for transitioning patients to buprenorphine from an opioid agonist, be it methadone or heroin. In this strategy, "microdoses" of buprenorphine (0.2–0.5 mg) are introduced, then gradually increased without waiting for withdrawal to start. Microinduction is based on the theory that multiple small doses of buprenorphine, given its high receptor affinity, will gradually replace the lower-affinity opioid already occupying the mu receptor sites. This slower change from full to partial agonist causes a less dramatic physiological shift, and hence fewer withdrawal symptoms. In contrast, a single large dose of buprenorphine will quickly replace the opioid and result in a sudden drop in agonist signaling.

This literature review examined 18 reports (n=63) of various buprenorphine microinduction strategies. The individual studies were quite heterogeneous, varying in opioid agonists, buprenorphine dosing, and time course. They all started with very low doses of buprenorphine (0.2–0.5 mg) and increased this dose slowly over time (from three to 112 days). Most transitioned over four to eight days and stabilized patients on daily doses of 8–16 mg of buprenorphine. Some utilized symptomatic treatment with clonidine during the induction period.

In most cases, the opioid agonist was continued while buprenorphine was being introduced and was later tapered over time or discontinued when the buprenorphine dose was judged adequate. Six studies used a different approach, choosing instead to utilize a transdermal patch, given its ability to consistently deliver small amounts of medication. These patches (buprenorphine in all cases but one in which fentanyl was used) served as a bridge from full agonist to eventual higher doses of sublingual buprenorphine. In most but not all of these cases, the previous opioid was discontinued when the transdermal patch was started.

RESULTS:

The review highlighted a few situations in which microinduction might be particularly beneficial, namely when transitioning to buprenorphine from methadone, and for patients with chronic pain.

The long half-life of methadone makes for a long withdrawal period when utilizing the traditional buprenorphine induction approach. Patients in this study were transitioned from methadone doses as high as 200 mg without requiring prior decrease of dose. Patients hospitalized for medical or surgical conditions could transition from illicit opioids without withdrawal. Individuals with chronic pain were transitioned without having to endure an increase in pain during the opioid withdrawal period.

CARLAT TAKE:
Before we all jump to microinductions for all our patients, there are caveats to consider. All of these papers were case reports or case series, excepting one open-label trial. Most did not evaluate withdrawal with validated measures. There is no standard protocol for microinduction, and no randomized trials compare microinduction to the usual method of induction. Nevertheless, this review shows the promise of this technique as an alternative for safe, effective initiation of buprenorphine treatment.

PRACTICE IMPLICATIONS:
While still relatively experimental, microinduction of buprenorphine could be considered for patients transitioning from methadone, using illicit opioids, or with chronic pain.

TABLE: Illustrative Buprenorphine Microdosing Protocol

Day	Buprenorphine Dosage	Preexisting Opioid Dosage (eg, methadone, heroin, fentanyl, etc.)
1	0.5 mg[1] once	Full dosage
2	0.5 mg BID	Full dosage
3	1 mg BID	Full dosage
4	2 mg BID	Full dosage
5	2 mg TID	Full dosage
6	2 mg QID	Full dosage
7	4 mg TID	STOP

Start 0.5 mg buprenorphine; patient can continue opioid agonist use. Gradually increase buprenorphine dose as tolerated until the patient reaches 8–12 mg of buprenorphine, then stop opioid agonist and titrate buprenorphine until patient no longer is experiencing cravings.

[1] Small doses can be obtained by cutting 2 mg strips into sections. One quarter of a strip provides 0.5 mg; one half of a strip provides 1 mg.

Gabapentin for Alcohol Use Disorder, Redux

REVIEW OF: Anton RF, Latham P, Voronin K, et al. Efficacy of gabapentin for the treatment of alcohol use disorder in patients with alcohol withdrawal symptoms: A randomized clinical trial. *JAMA Intern Med.* 2020;180(5):728–736.

STUDY TYPE: Randomized controlled trial

GABAPENTIN HAS HAD mixed results in the treatment of alcohol use disorder (AUD), but it is clearly effective in the treatment of alcohol withdrawal syndrome (AWS). In this study, researchers tested whether gabapentin might be effective in treating adults with AUD who also have a history of AWS.

The investigators conducted a 16-week randomized controlled trial comparing gabapentin to placebo. Ninety patients with AUD and a history of AWS were enrolled (44 in the gabapentin arm, 46 in the placebo arm). Here, AWS was defined as a self-reported history of withdrawal symptoms; however, those with a history of withdrawal seizures were excluded.

Participants were ages 18–70, 94% were White, and 77% were men. They drank a mean of 86% of pretreatment days, with 83% being heavy drinking days (defined as five or more drinks per day for men and four or more drinks per day for women). They were required to have been abstinent for three days prior to randomization. The study took place in an academic medical center and was sponsored by the National Institute on Alcohol Abuse and Alcoholism.

Gabapentin was started at 300 mg at bedtime and titrated over five days to 300 mg in the morning, 300 mg at noon, and 600 mg at bedtime. Patients received nine 20-minute medical management visits. The primary outcome was the percentage of participants with no heavy drinking days.

RESULTS:

After 16 weeks, more gabapentin-treated individuals had no heavy drinking days compared with placebo (27% vs 9%; p=0.02), with a number needed to treat (NNT) of 5.4. More gabapentin-treated patients also achieved total abstinence compared to placebo (18% vs 4%; p=0.04), with an NNT of 6.2. The effect was more pronounced for patients with histories of more severe withdrawal. Among those who had reported less severe withdrawal, there was no difference between gabapentin and placebo. Dizziness was reported more often in the gabapentin arm versus the placebo arm (57% vs 33%; p=0.02), but no serious adverse events were reported.

CARLAT TAKE:

For patients with AUD and a history of AWS, gabapentin was associated with more patients having no heavy drinking days and continued abstinence. However, this trial did not address the effects of gabapentin beyond four months of use. In some states, gabapentin is a controlled substance, and there are concerns regarding its misuse, addictive potential, and interaction with other sedating substances.

PRACTICE IMPLICATIONS:
For patients with a history of withdrawal who struggle with AUD, gabapentin may be helpful after first-line options like naltrexone and acamprosate have been exhausted.

Internet-Based Approaches for Gambling Problems

REVIEW OF: Sagoe D, Griffiths MD, Erevik EK, et al. Internet-based treatment of gambling problems: A systematic review and meta-analysis of randomized controlled trials. *J Behav Addict.* 2021;10(3):546–565.

STUDY TYPE: Systematic review and meta-analysis

Problematic gambling is common, affecting up to 6.5% of all adults. But only 10% of them get treated, at least in part due to limited provider availability and stigma. The easy access and anonymity offered by internet-based gambling treatment programs address both barriers—but how well do these programs work?

Researchers conducted a systematic review and meta-analysis, compiling 13 randomized trials that enrolled over 2,000 participants. Eight of the studies had control groups, the specifics of which varied between trials. Overall, 22 treatments were tested; 13 of them were based on cognitive behavioral therapy, while the others were based on a range of other psychotherapeutic interventions (motivational interviewing, couples therapy, and brief advice, among others). The number of sessions ranged from one to 28 (mean 9.9 sessions), and four of the protocols included therapist support. The outcomes were gambling frequency, amount of money lost, and score on a gambling severity scale (different studies used different scales), which the authors called "general gambling symptoms."

RESULTS:

Internet-based treatments were associated with improved outcomes, particularly for general gambling symptoms. At the conclusion of treatment, the effect size (Hedges' g) for improvement of general gambling symptoms was 0.729 (95% CI [0.43, 1.03]), indicating a medium to large effect. The effect sizes for gambling frequency (g=0.29; 95% CI [0.14, 0.45]) and amount of money lost (g=0.19; 95% CI [0.11, 0.27]) were more modest.

Ten of the studies included assessments after a follow-up period (ranging from one to 36 months, mean 8.3 months), and these showed that benefits persisted over time for general gambling symptoms (g=1.20; 95% CI [0.79, 1.61]), gambling frequency (g=0.36; 95% CI [0.12, 0.60]), and amount of money lost (g=0.20; 95% CI [0.12, 0.29]).

Patients with more severe symptoms tended to show a greater degree of improvement, and interventions that included therapist support were associated with a greater benefit. Unsurprisingly, studies that included a control group typically had smaller effect sizes. The authors compared these results with previous findings and determined that internet-based treatments did not work quite as well as in-person therapy but did work better than self-guided interventions (Goslar M et al, *J Behav Addict* 2017;6(2):142–162).

CARLAT TAKE:
This study shows us that internet-based gambling treatments can be effective.

PRACTICE IMPLICATIONS:
For patients with gambling disorder who prefer anonymity or online treatment, or lack access to a therapist, consider internet-based treatment. A variety of methods and protocols are likely to be effective.

Is AA the Toast of the Town?

REVIEW OF: Kelly JF, Humphreys K, Ferri M. Alcoholics Anonymous and other 12-step programs for alcohol use disorder. *Cochrane Database Syst Rev.* 2020;3(3):CD012880.

STUDY TYPE: Systematic review and meta-analysis

Alcoholics Anonymous (AA) is the most widely used psychosocial treatment for alcohol use disorder (AUD). Twelve-step facilitation (TSF) is a professionally delivered treatment that facilitates involvement in AA. It is an active, ongoing methodology—not a one-time referral or a pamphlet. Historically, the low quality of available evidence has limited our ability to speak confidently of AA's effectiveness. Previous Cochrane reviews (which tend to occupy the highest rung on the evidence pyramid) have concluded that superiority cannot be assumed for AA over other therapies (Ferri M et al, *Cochrane Database Syst Rev* 2006;(3):CD005032).

So it caused a stir in the substance use treatment community when Kelly et al reported in an updated 2020 Cochrane review that manualized AA/TSF programs are more or equally effective for various AUD-related outcomes than psychological clinical interventions, including cognitive behavioral therapy (CBT), motivational enhancement therapy (MET), and other 12-step variants.

In Cochrane fashion, the authors scoured the world's literature for interventional trials (randomized, quasi-experimental, and non-randomized) that compared AA/TSF to something else (CBT or MET, 12-step variants, or no treatment). They also searched for economic studies that assessed health care savings. The authors identified 27 studies that in total included 10,565 participants.

RESULTS:

Compared to other clinical interventions, manualized AA/TSF produced higher rates of continuous abstinence at 12 months (risk ratio 1.21; 95% CI [1.03, 1.42]). This effect was consistent at 24 and 36 months. Manualized AA/TSF performed equally well or slightly better than other clinical interventions on all other measures of sobriety (eg, longest period of abstinence, percentage of days abstinent, and drinking intensity outcomes). Non-manualized AA/TSF performed as well as other clinical interventions on all primary and secondary outcomes.

Regarding the economic outcomes, four of five studies found substantial cost savings in favor of AA/TSF. Kelly told the *New York Times*, "It's the closest thing in public health we have to a free lunch" (Frakt A and Carroll AE. *New York Times.* March 11, 2020).

CARLAT TAKE:
Although studies that assess the impact of AA/TSF are heterogeneous—as is AA, which is part of its strength—this Cochrane meta-analysis was able to confirm the utility of AA/TSF, which has helped millions of people for over 80 years.

PRACTICE IMPLICATIONS:

Patients with AUD are likely to benefit from AA/TSF referrals. The National Institute on Alcohol Abuse and Alcoholism has published a guide for clinical and research settings (https://pubs.niaaa.nih.gov/publications/projectmatch/match01.pdf). Successful engagement appears to stimulate AA attendance and involvement, which in turn enhances sobriety.

Meds for Alcohol Use Disorder

REVIEW OF: Heikkinen M, Taipale H, Tanskanen A, Mittendorfer-Rutz E, Lähteenvuo M, Tiihonen J. Real-world effectiveness of pharmacological treatments of alcohol use disorders in a Swedish nation-wide cohort of 125 556 patients. *Addiction*. 2021;116(8):1990–1998.

STUDY TYPE: Prospective cohort study

In the US, only 9% of patients diagnosed with alcohol use disorder (AUD) are prescribed AUD medication (Kranzler HR and Soyka M, *JAMA* 2018;320(8):815–824). This study compared the real-world impact of four medications, three of which—disulfiram, naltrexone, and acamprosate—are FDA approved for AUD.

Researchers used national databases in Sweden to identify 125,556 people (62.5% men) ages 16–64 with a diagnosis of AUD and followed them prospectively for 10 years. They excluded individuals with schizophrenia or bipolar disorder. The researchers recorded whether participants picked up prescriptions for naltrexone, disulfiram, acamprosate, or nalmefene (an opioid antagonist like naltrexone that is only available for opioid use disorder in the US). Their primary outcome was hospitalization due to AUD.

RESULTS:

Naltrexone was associated with reduced rates of hospitalization, both as a monotherapy and when combined with disulfiram or acamprosate. For hospitalizations due to alcohol-related causes, naltrexone monotherapy decreased rates by 11%, naltrexone + acamprosate decreased rates by 26%, and naltrexone + disulfiram decreased rates by 24%. The results were nearly identical for all-cause hospitalization.

One big surprise was that acamprosate alone was associated with an increased risk of hospitalization. Disulfiram and nalmefene monotherapy were not associated with significantly different rates of hospitalization.

Finally, researchers found that benzodiazepines were associated with both an 18% increased hospitalization rate due to AUD and an 11% higher mortality rate. While this result is not unexpected, it does emphasize the dangers of prescribing benzos to patients who are actively drinking or diagnosed with AUD.

CARLAT TAKE:

At first glance, it may seem that naltrexone in combination with another medication is the best option. But the authors pointed out that even though combinations outperformed naltrexone monotherapy, patients who received combination medication may also have been more likely to be receiving care from specialists. Potentially, other factors related to the specialists' care might have been responsible for the lower hospitalization rates. The authors speculated that acamprosate's poor efficacy may partially be explained by the fact that it requires dosing three times daily; adherence may have been poorer in the acamprosate arm than for other medications. But why this would be associated with worse outcomes than no medication at all is unclear.

PRACTICE IMPLICATIONS:

Consider naltrexone, both alone or alongside disulfiram or acamprosate, for patients with AUD—and whenever possible, avoid benzodiazepines.

A Novel Treatment for Methamphetamine Use Disorder

REVIEW OF: Trivedi MH, Walker R, Ling W, et al. Bupropion and naltrexone in methamphetamine use disorder. *N Engl J Med.* 2021;384(2):140–153.

STUDY TYPE: Randomized, double-blind, placebo-controlled trial with sequential parallel comparison design

METHAMPHETAMINE USE DISORDER is increasingly a cause of overdose deaths in the U.S. Pharmacologic options to treat methamphetamine use disorder are scarce, but pilot studies suggest that bupropion and naltrexone may be effective, either alone or in combination, and this study tested them in combination.

The authors designed this double-blind, randomized, placebo-controlled study in two phases. First, patients were randomized to treatment or placebo for six weeks, with three times as many assigned to placebo. In the second stage, patients who responded to placebo were removed, and the remaining placebo subjects were re-randomized to either more placebo or active treatment for another six weeks, this time with equal numbers in the placebo and treatment arms. The point of this design was to dampen the placebo response in the second phase of the study.

The subjects were adults with moderate to severe methamphetamine use disorder who wanted to quit or reduce use, recruited through advertisements and direct referrals. On average, they had used methamphetamine on 27 of the previous 30 days. The active combo treatment was extended-release (ER) naltrexone 380 mg intramuscular every three weeks (a relatively high dose) and ER bupropion 450 mg daily.

There were 403 participants in stage one, and 225 who did not respond to placebo were re-randomized to stage two. Overall retention was good (77.4%). The primary outcome was response, defined as one out of four urine tests negative for methamphetamine in the last two weeks of stage one or stage two.

RESULTS:

Naltrexone-bupropion was significantly more effective than placebo. The weighted average response was 13.6% for the active group and 2.5% for placebo (p<0.001), and the number needed to treat (NNT) was 9. Adverse events, such as nausea, vomiting, and constipation, were evenly divided between active and placebo conditions.

CARLAT TAKE:

Naltrexone-bupropion combination is somewhat effective for methamphetamine use disorder. While the NNT of 9 is not fantastic, this treatment was backed by a well-designed trial, and in a disorder with such devastating consequences, every tool is important.

PRACTICE IMPLICATIONS:
Consider naltrexone-bupropion in combination with your usual nonpharmaceutical treatment recommendations for methamphetamine use disorder—but don't expect every patient to respond.

Opioid Agonist Treatment and Decreased Mortality

REVIEW OF: Santo T Jr, Clark B, Hickman M, et al. Association of opioid agonist treatment with all-cause mortality and specific causes of death among people with opioid dependence: A systematic review and meta-analysis. *JAMA Psychiatry.* 2021;78(9):979–993. [Published correction appears in *JAMA Psychiatry* 2022;79(5):516]

STUDY TYPE: Systematic review and meta-analysis

It has been well established that opioid agonist treatment (OAT) saves lives by reducing rates of fatal drug overdose. But OAT can reduce mortality in other ways as well. In this study, researchers analyzed data from 15 randomized clinical trials and 36 cohort studies across nearly 750,000 participants to conduct an unprecedented examination of the association of OAT, specifically methadone and buprenorphine, with various causes of death among patients with opioid use disorder (OUD).

RESULTS:

As expected, the authors found that OAT was associated with an impressive reduction in all-cause mortality; patients receiving OAT died less than half as often as those not receiving OAT (risk ratio [RR] 0.47; 95% CI [0.42, 0.53]). This reduction in risk of all-cause mortality was the same whether patients were taking methadone or buprenorphine. It was also consistent across a host of patient characteristics including age, gender, HIV or hepatitis C viral status, and whether the patient used drugs intravenously.

Researchers found that patients receiving OAT had a decreased mortality due to several specific causes of death as well. They had not only a two-thirds reduced risk of unintentional drug overdose (RR 0.35; 95% CI [0.27, 0.46]), but also a reduced risk of death due to suicide (RR 0.48; 95% CI [0.37, 0.61]), cancer (RR 0.72; 95% CI [0.54, 0.98]), alcohol (RR 0.59; 95% CI [0.49, 0.72]), and cardiovascular conditions (RR 0.69; 95% CI [0.60, 0.79]).

The six studies specifically looking at OAT outcomes in and around incarceration were particularly striking. The single study of OAT during incarceration showed a large decrease in the risk of all-cause (RR 0.24; 95% CI [0.12, 0.47]) and drug- or suicide-related death (RR 0.17; 95% CI [0.05, 0.57]). Similarly, three studies showed dramatic reductions in risk of all-cause (RR 0.24; 95% CI [0.15, 0.37]) and drug-related (RR 0.19; 95% CI [0.10, 0.37]) deaths in the first four weeks after release for those who initiated OAT while incarcerated, compared to those who didn't.

Researchers noted two caveats, neither one unexpected. First, and most obviously, OAT must be taken to be effective. Patients became particularly vulnerable if they discontinued treatment, with all-cause mortality increasing six-fold in the first month (RR 6.01; 95% CI [4.32, 8.36]) and remaining nearly double (RR 1.81; 95% CI [1.50, 2.18]) for as long as they were not receiving OAT. In addition, all-cause mortality and drug-related poisoning were twice as high during the first month of methadone treatment (RR 2.01; 95% CI [1.55, 5.09]) compared to the rest of the time on OAT. This may be related to the gradual titration of methadone during treatment initiation, which can potentially leave patients vulnerable while still on a low dose. Buprenorphine can be titrated much more quickly, which is likely why this trend was not observed among those receiving buprenorphine.

CARLAT TAKE:
OAT is a powerful tool for reducing death due to a variety of causes in patients with OUD. This trend is consistent across demographic groups and is especially pronounced during and upon release from incarceration. Mortality increases when OAT is discontinued, particularly in the first month.

PRACTICE IMPLICATIONS:
Recommend OAT to patients suffering from OUD. Your risk/benefit discussion might include a reduced risk of all-cause mortality and the importance of treatment adherence.

ADDICTION PSYCHIATRY

Should Prolonged Abstinence From Alcohol Be Required Before Liver Transplant?

REVIEW OF: Herrick-Reynolds KM, Punchhi G, Greenberg RS, et al. Evaluation of early vs standard liver transplant for alcohol-associated liver disease. *JAMA Surg.* 2021;156(11):1026–1034.

STUDY TYPE: Retrospective cohort study

TRADITIONALLY, PATIENTS WITH alcohol-related liver disease are told that they have to be sober for at least six months before they can have a liver transplant (LT). There aren't enough transplantable livers to go around, and patients have been held to this abstinence requirement to demonstrate that they are committed to sobriety and less likely to damage a recently transplanted liver. The authors of this study wanted to find out if this practice is warranted by comparing outcomes between two groups of patients: those who received LT before six months of sobriety versus after.

Authors retrospectively looked at patients with alcohol-related liver disease who had received LT between October 2012 and November 2020 and divided them into two groups: The early LT group had less than 180 days of abstinence at the time of transplant, and the standard LT group had greater than 180 days. Outcomes included patient survival, early relapse (drinking within 90 days of LT), relapse-free survival, and hazardous relapse–free survival. Hazardous relapse was defined as binge drinking (five or more drinks for men, or four or more drinks for women), at-risk drinking (14 or more drinks for men per week, or seven or more drinks for women per week), or frequent drinking (four or more occasions per week).

Of 163 patients, 88 received early LT and 75 received standard LT. 66% of the patients were male, 34% were female, and 87% were White; sex and race did not differ significantly between the two groups. The two significant demographic differences were that patients who underwent early LT were younger (49.7 years old vs 54.6 years old) and had more severe illness (Model for End-Stage Liver Disease [MELD] score 35 vs 20) compared to patients in the standard LT group. At the time of transplant, the mean number of days abstinent in the early LT group was 66.5 days vs 481 days in the standard LT group.

RESULTS:

One-year and three-year survival rates were similar for both groups (94.1% for early LT vs 95.9% for standard LT at one year; 83% for early LT vs 78.6% for standard LT at three years). Relapse-free survival and hazardous relapse–free survival rates were also comparable at one year and three years. Early LT had no association with relapse or hazardous relapse.

The researchers did find an association between younger age and return to drinking. Patients younger than 60 were more likely to have a relapse (adjusted hazard ratio [aHR] 8.31; p=0.008) or a hazardous relapse (aHR 9.02; p=0.009) compared to those older than 60. Unsurprisingly, researchers also found that patients who had an early relapse had lower overall survival (aHR 5.46; p=0.02).

CARLAT TAKE:
In this study, LT outcomes were similar for patients with alcohol-related liver disease whether they were abstinent for six months prior to surgery or not, suggesting that this traditional waiting period is arbitrary.

PRACTICE IMPLICATIONS:
Advocate for patients with alcohol use disorder to receive LT early if they're being asked to wait.

Smoking Cessation Intervention for Hospitalized Patients

REVIEW OF: Brown RA, Minami H, Hecht J, et al. Sustained care smoking cessation intervention for individuals hospitalized for psychiatric disorders: The Helping HAND 3 randomized clinical trial. *JAMA Psychiatry.* 2021;78(8):839–847. [Published correction appears in *JAMA Psychiatry* 2022;79(1):87]

STUDY TYPE: Randomized controlled trial

Adults with serious mental illness (SMI) tend to smoke heavily and die at much younger ages than the general population. Smoking is forbidden in most psychiatric hospitals, so patients become abstinent during their inpatient stays and usually manage their withdrawal symptoms with nicotine replacement therapy (NRT). However, most patients resume smoking soon after discharge.

The authors of this study reasoned that the forced abstinence during patients' hospital stays could jump-start efforts to promote smoking cessation after discharge. They compared treatment as usual (TAU), consisting of NRT patches and smoking cessation information, to a systematic approach called sustained care (SC). The main components of SC are a pre-discharge motivational interviewing session; NRT patches on discharge; post-discharge cessation counseling via phone, text, or internet; and post-discharge automated interactive calls or texts.

This National Institute of Mental Health–funded study took place in a private psychiatric hospital in Austin, Texas. Adults who smoked more than five cigarettes a day were randomized to TAU (n=173) or SC (n=169). Subjects smoked an average of 17 cigarettes per day at baseline. The most common discharge diagnoses were depression, substance-related disorders, bipolar disorder, and schizophrenia. Hospital length of stay averaged six days. Two-thirds of subjects were economically disadvantaged (household annual income less than $25,000)—a factor that, in addition to SMI, is known to contribute to lower success with smoking cessation.

The main outcome measure was smoking abstinence for the past seven days, verified by salivary detection of a nicotine metabolite called cotinine. Because both NRT and cigarettes can produce cotinine, exhaled carbon monoxide was measured in subjects who reported recent NRT use. Subjects were followed at one, three, and six months post-discharge, and their use of smoking cessation treatments (eg, counseling, NRT, bupropion, varenicline) was recorded.

RESULTS:

The SC group was significantly more likely to be abstinent than the TAU group at six months (8.9% and 3.5%, respectively; p=0.01). The SC group was also significantly more likely (75% vs 41%; p<0.001) to use smoking cessation treatments in the six months following discharge.

CARLAT TAKE:
This intervention shows that adults with SMI can be successfully engaged in smoking cessation treatment following hospital discharge.

PRACTICE IMPLICATIONS:
Smoking cessation interventions for psychiatrically hospitalized patients are more likely to succeed if they include not just NRT, but also motivational interviewing and post-discharge follow-up.

Starting Buprenorphine: Is Timing Everything?

REVIEW OF: Jakubowski A, Lu T, DiRenno F, et al. Same-day vs. delayed buprenorphine prescribing and patient retention in an office-based buprenorphine treatment program. *J Subst Abuse Treat*. 2020;119:108140.

STUDY TYPE: Retrospective cohort study

Buprenorphine is a safe and effective treatment of opioid use disorder (OUD), but studies show that less than two-thirds of patients treated with buprenorphine are still in treatment six months later (Timko C et al, *J Addict Dis* 2016;35(1):22–35). Since the highest rate of dropout is during the first month of treatment, Jakubowski and colleagues decided to look at factors affecting dropout and hypothesized that the timing of the first dose of buprenorphine might be a decisive factor. The researchers speculated that patients receiving their first dose on their very first visit might be more likely to stay in treatment over time.

The investigators looked retrospectively at a cohort of 222 patients engaged in buprenorphine treatment at a federally qualified health center. They divided the patients into two groups: those who were prescribed buprenorphine at the initial evaluation, and those who were prescribed buprenorphine later, but within 30 days of the initial visit. Treatment consisted of buprenorphine prescription plus visits with a primary care physician every one to two weeks until stable, and then monthly.

RESULTS:

Of the 222 patients, 89 (40%) were prescribed buprenorphine on the same day as the initial visit and 133 patients (60%) were prescribed it later within the first 30 days. Eighty percent of patients remained in treatment through the first 30 days. A higher percentage (85% vs 77%) of same-day prescription patients remained in treatment through the first 30 days, but this difference was not statistically significant (p=0.11). Researchers noted that alcohol or benzodiazepine use was associated with delayed prescription of buprenorphine, but the results were the same even when these factors were adjusted for.

CARLAT TAKE:
This study did not identify a statistically significant improvement in treatment retention associated with initiating buprenorphine on the first day of evaluation compared to later initiation.

PRACTICE IMPLICATIONS:
It's reasonable to consider induction with buprenorphine on the same day you evaluate a patient for OUD, but delaying for a reasonable period for sound clinical reasons isn't likely to harm patients.

Stigmatizing Smoking: An Effective Deterrent?

REVIEW OF: Cortland CI, Shapiro JR, Guzman IY, Ray LA. The ironic effects of stigmatizing smoking: Combining stereotype threat theory with behavioral pharmacology. *Addiction.* 2019;114(10):1842–1848.

STUDY TYPE: Randomized controlled trial

Tobacco use is the single most preventable cause of death, disease, and disability in the United States. The American government spends $50 million each year on tobacco cessation efforts, including many public service campaigns that attempt to shame or stigmatize smoking as an undesirable behavior. This study investigates how the social stereotype threat—creating concern that one will be judged unfavorably by others—may impact one's ability to resist the next cigarette.

In this randomized controlled trial, 77 non-treatment-seeking, otherwise-healthy adult smokers were recruited from the community and randomized to either receive a stereotype threat or a control message after 12 hours of abstinence. Specifically, the stereotype threat group was told that the investigators were interested in "whether non-smokers are superior across all positive traits or only certain types [such as] willpower, laziness, weakness and responsibility," bringing to participants' minds the negative stereotypes of people who smoke. Both the intervention group and the control group were given a lighter, an ashtray, some of their favorite cigarettes, and a small monetary reward for delaying smoking during hour-long observation periods.

RESULTS:

The investigators found no significant difference in time-to-smoke data between groups. However, when they controlled for baseline latency-to-smoke, they found that the stereotype threat was associated with lesser latency-to-smoke (hazard ratio 0.50; 95% CI [0.30, 0.85]). The researchers concluded that the stereotype threat actually functioned as a "smoking-promoting message."

Major limitations of the study included generalizability to the real world, including observing the participants for one hour and the simplicity of the stereotype threat, which may not replicate the complex nature of stereotypes in specific communities and in society. Another major limitation was that the control group did not receive a non-stigmatizing, smoking-related cue.

CARLAT TAKE:
While it doesn't readily approximate the complex nature of stereotypes or stigma, this study suggests that shaming people may increase their likelihood of lighting up.

PRACTICE IMPLICATIONS:
Doing no harm means avoiding stigmatizing patients who suffer from nicotine (and likely all) addiction.

ADDICTION PSYCHIATRY

Sublocade vs SL Buprenorphine After Release From Jail

REVIEW OF: Lee JD, Malone M, McDonald R, et al. Comparison of treatment retention of adults with opioid addiction managed with extended-release buprenorphine vs daily sublingual buprenorphine-naloxone at time of release from jail. *JAMA Netw Open*. 2021;4(9):e2123032.

STUDY TYPE: Randomized comparative-effectiveness trial

When people with opioid use disorder (OUD) are released from incarceration, they have a high risk of overdose—especially if they are not prescribed any medication for OUD (MOUD). We know that methadone, sublingual buprenorphine/naloxone (SL-BUP), and injectable naltrexone all improve OUD outcomes in this population. What about the relatively new extended-release buprenorphine formulation (XR-BUP; brand name Sublocade)? In this study, researchers compared SL-BUP with XR-BUP to assess feasibility and acceptability among people being released from incarceration.

Researchers enrolled 52 incarcerated, soon-to-be-released adults from New York City jails who were already receiving SL-BUP for OUD. Half were randomized to start XR-BUP in prison with the goal of continuing it in the community. All participants were followed for eight weeks post-release. The primary clinical outcome was treatment retention.

RESULTS:

The researchers first examined whether it was even feasible to give XR-BUP injections in incarceration settings, concluding that it was. Most participants (21/26) received at least one dose before release (mean number of doses 2.3). Those on the XR-BUP injection required fewer daily prison clinic visits than those prescribed SL-BUP. XR-BUP participants also were unable to divert their medication; there were two incidents of diversion in the SL-BUP group. This led researchers to conclude that starting XR-BUP while incarcerated saves time and labor compared to SL-BUP.

XR-BUP was superior to SL-BUP on several post-release clinical outcomes. It was associated with a two-fold increase in treatment retention at week eight (69% vs 35%), the average length of time that patients stayed on buprenorphine after release was higher (6.1 vs 2.6 weeks), and there were more opioid-free urine drug tests (55.4% vs 38.5%). No differences in rates of serious adverse events were observed between the two groups, and there were no overdoses observed in study participants.

The researchers did identify a few barriers to XR-BUP, including lack of knowledge about the new formulation, perceived lack of access in the community, opposition to needlesticks, and a preference for staying with the familiar SL formulation. At the conclusion of the study, seven XR-BUP participants chose to switch back to SL-BUP, citing injection pain and personal preference.

CARLAT TAKE:

XR-BUP appears to be a very promising intervention for this high-risk population. A 2022 retrospective cohort study of incarcerated individuals (n=54) in Rhode Island augmented these findings, finding that 61% of those released on XR-BUP engaged in MOUD, of which 30% continued XR-BUP (Martin RA et al, *J Subst Abuse Treat* 2022;142:108851).

PRACTICE IMPLICATIONS:

Expanding access to XR-BUP in correctional settings by making it more available and educating patients and clinicians will likely improve outcomes for those suffering from OUD.

Suboxone vs Vivitrol for Opioid Use Disorder

REVIEW OF: Nunes EV Jr, Scodes JM, Pavlicova M, et al. Sublingual buprenorphine-naloxone compared with injection naltrexone for opioid use disorder: Potential utility of patient characteristics in guiding choice of treatment. *Am J Psychiatry.* 2021;178(7):660–671.

STUDY TYPE: Post-hoc analysis of randomized comparative-effectiveness trial data

For decades, methadone and buprenorphine-naloxone (BUP) have been the gold standards for opioid use disorder (OUD), with naltrexone largely considered second line. However, that wisdom was challenged by a pair of landmark studies showing the non-inferiority of long-acting injectable naltrexone (XR-NTX) as compared to sublingual BUP (Lee JD et al, *Lancet* 2018;10118(27):309–318; Tanum L et al, *JAMA Psych* 2017;74(12):1197–1205). These papers showed that the treatments are equally effective for those patients who manage to start treatment. However, patients are much more likely to tolerate starting treatment with BUP because induction only requires 12 hours of abstinence from opioids. In contrast, patients must be opioid-free for at least seven days before they can start XR-NTX—a tall order for many people with OUD.

Hoping to better understand which patients might do better with BUP versus XR-NTX, Nunes et al reexamined data from one of the aforementioned trials (Lee et al, 2018). In this trial, 287 patients with OUD were randomized to BUP (8–24 mg sublingual daily) and 283 patients were randomized to XR-NTX (380 mg intramuscular every 28 days). Participants were assessed weekly with urine drug screens and self-reported substance use. Authors examined the data for demographic characteristics predictive of successful medication initiation and rate of returning to use.

RESULTS:

Overall, it was easier for participants to successfully start BUP (5.9% failure rate) compared to XR-NTX (27.9% failure rate). Participants with moderate to severe chronic pain had a much higher failure rate with XR-NTX compared to BUP (32.44% vs 1.99%; odds ratio [OR] 23.68; 95% CI [8.21, 68.34]). This finding has face validity: Chronic pain likely makes it difficult to stop opioids for several days vs 12 hours. Individuals randomized to XR-NTX soon after their last opioid use (less than three days) had a higher rate of treatment failure compared to BUP (41.30% vs 1.45%; OR 47.79; 95% CI [11.15, 204.89]). This is also no surprise: Use of naltrexone soon after opioid use may trigger withdrawal symptoms. Participants who stated a preference for BUP also had a much lower failure rate if they received BUP than if they received XR-NTX (0.88% vs 33.01%; OR 55.28; 95% CI [7.27, 420.15]). Those who stated a neutral preference for receiving BUP also had a much lower failure rate if randomized to BUP compared to XR-NTX (23.62% vs 3.25%; OR 9.22; 95% CI [3.35, 25.39]), while those who disagreed with having a preference for BUP had similar failure rates with both medications.

On the other hand, being on probation or parole tended to predict success with XR-NTX compared to the study participants overall. In this group, XR-NTX had a similar failure-to-initiate rate as BUP (17.39% vs 14.39%; OR 1.25; 95% CI [0.42, 3.61]). XR-NTX also had an edge among homeless individuals, for whom the rate of returning to opioid use was lower with XR-NTX as compared to BUP (41.44% vs 68.64%; OR 0.32; 95% CI [0.15, 0.68]). This is the only patient characteristic that was predictive of 24-week relapse, as opposed to failure to initiate treatment, for which homelessness was not a significant moderator.

CARLAT TAKE:

It should be noted that only opioid-related outcomes were measured, and that potentially relevant outcomes unrelated to opioid use were not reported. For example, a patient with comorbid alcohol use disorder (AUD) might fare better with XR-NTX, since it is an effective medication for both AUD and OUD. XR-NTX might also be preferred for patients with comorbid benzodiazepine use disorder, since BUP and benzos can produce fatal respiratory suppression when combined.

PRACTICE IMPLICATIONS:

This study largely confirms previous findings that BUP and XR-NTX are both effective treatments for OUD once started, but that BUP is easier to initiate than XR-NTX. Factors predicting better success with initiating BUP include chronic pain, recent opioid use, and preference for BUP. Initiation of BUP and XR-NTX fared similarly for patients on probation. Homeless patients had lower rates of return to use with XR-NTX. These data provide useful guidance, but other patient factors should still be considered when making a final medication choice.

CHILD AND ADOLESCENT PSYCHIATRY

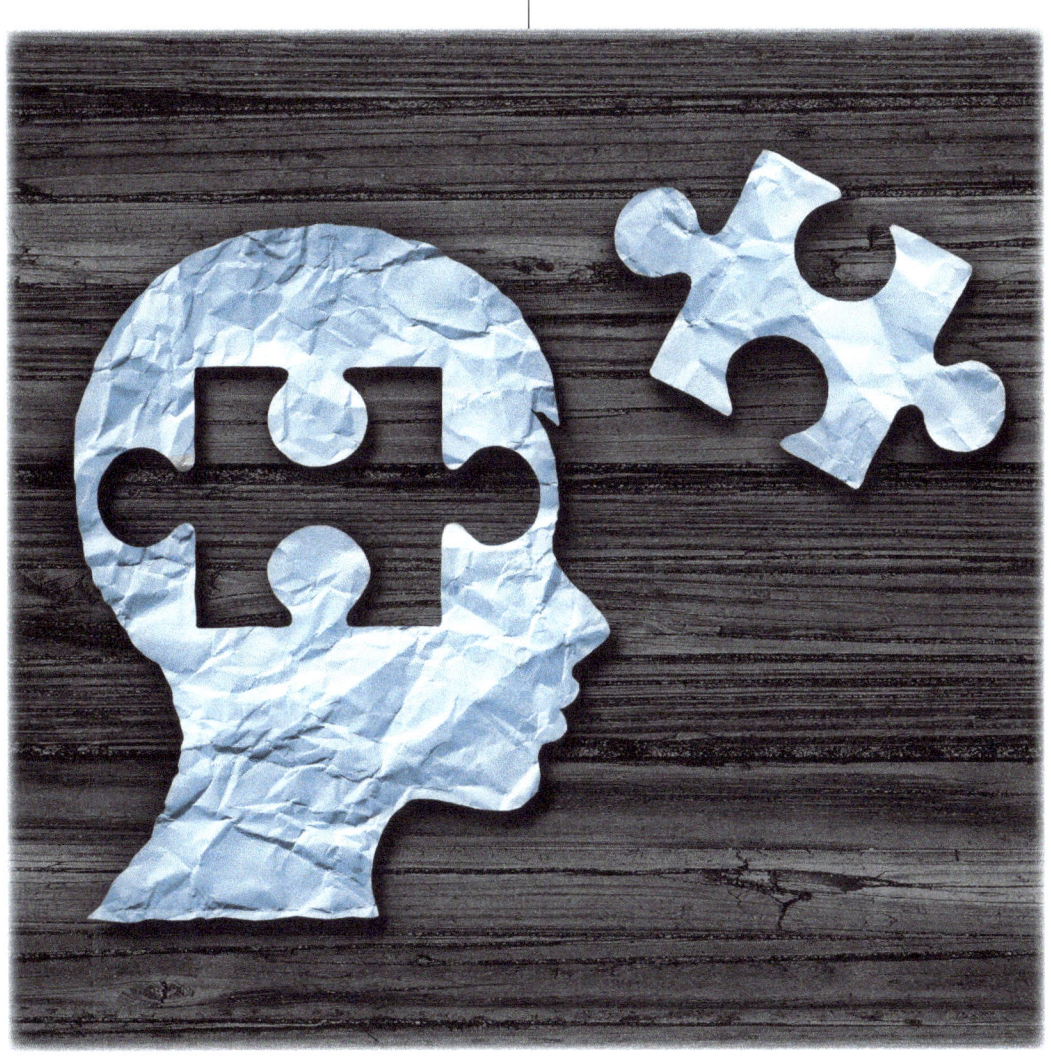

ADHD Prevalence in Black American Children

REVIEW OF: Cénat JM, Blais-Rochette C, Morse C, et al. Prevalence and risk factors associated with attention-deficit/hyperactivity disorder among US Black individuals: A systematic review and meta-analysis. *JAMA Psychiatry.* 2021;78(1):21–28.

STUDY TYPE: Systematic review and meta-analysis

In the general population, the reported prevalence of ADHD is about 10%, with estimates varying from around 5% to 15%. However, Black people are usually underrepresented in these (and other) studies. Estimates of ADHD in the Black population are less precise, with an estimated prevalence of 5% to over 20%. This study tried to improve the accuracy of prevalence measures of ADHD among Black individuals, as well as identify specific risk factors for ADHD in this population.

The authors found 21 articles published between 1979 and 2019 with 24 independent samples or subsamples of American Black people. Most (13) included both children and adolescents. Eight samples included only children, one included only adolescents, and two included only adults.

RESULTS:

From these studies, the researchers conducted a meta-analysis and computed a pooled ADHD prevalence of 14.5% (95% CI [10.64%, 19.56%]). When only the samples of children and adolescents were included, the prevalence was 13.9%, which was not significantly different.

Older children (10–17 years) were more likely to receive an ADHD diagnosis, as were males. Males also received more prescriptions for ADHD than females. In at-risk populations like juvenile offenders, Black youth were less likely to be diagnosed with ADHD. Interestingly, Black parents were less likely to report ADHD symptoms in their children, while teachers reported more symptoms. Low socioeconomic status was a risk factor for ADHD in Black individuals, but high socioeconomic status was not a protective factor against ADHD (as it is in White individuals).

CARLAT TAKE:

This study shows that Black Americans are more likely to meet diagnostic criteria for ADHD than the general population, with a prevalence of about 14% vs about 10% in the general population. It's not clear what drives this disparity, although an increased tendency for teachers to identify ADHD symptoms in Black children, lower socioeconomic status, as well as culturally determined biases in the ADHD construct itself might be factors.

PRACTICE IMPLICATIONS:

These data contradict the DSM-5, which states that Black people have a lower rate of ADHD. It's a good reminder to screen all patients carefully and be aware of potential biases in diagnosis and in the literature.

Can Stimulants Prevent Crime?

REVIEW OF: Mohr-Jensen C, Müller Bisgaard C, Boldsen SK, Steinhausen HC. Attention-deficit/hyperactivity disorder in childhood and adolescence and the risk of crime in young adulthood in a Danish nationwide study. *J Am Acad Child Adolesc Psychiatry.* 2019;58(4):443–452.

STUDY TYPE: Case-control study

ADHD HAS LONG been linked to behaviors associated with arrest and incarceration. From traffic violations to violent crimes, children and young adults with ADHD are more likely to be charged than peers. Is ADHD causing these behaviors? And if ADHD is an independent risk factor for criminal behavior, can that risk be decreased with stimulants?

These big questions require population-based studies. Researchers evaluated data from Danish national medical and prescription registries, matching 4,231 children diagnosed with ADHD from 1995 to 2005 with controls based on sex and age. Follow-up data from an average of 22 years were obtained, including arrests, incarcerations, comorbid substance use disorders, time on stimulant medications, as well as psychosocial factors. In this study, nearly all of the stimulant prescriptions (98%) were for methylphenidate, and most of the children (85%) were male.

RESULTS:

After controlling for confounders such as psychiatric comorbidity, socioeconomic status, parental psychopathology, and other psychosocial factors, males with ADHD were 60% more likely (hazard ratio [HR] 1.6; 95% CI = [1.5, 1.8]) to be convicted of a crime and 70% more likely (HR 1.7; 95% CI = [1.5, 1.9]) to be incarcerated. For females, the effect was even more profound—120% more likely (HR 2.2) to be convicted and 190% more likely (HR 2.9; 95% CI = [1.6, 5.3]) to be incarcerated. However, when looking at times of active treatment with stimulant medications, the risk of conviction dropped significantly by 40% for both males and females (males: HR = 0.6; 95% CI = [0.6, 0.7]; females: HR = 0.6; 95% CI = [0.4, 0.9]), compared to time periods off medications. Incarceration risk also dropped by 40% (HR = 0.6; 95% CI = [0.5, 0.7]) for males, but not significantly for females.

CARLAT TAKE:

This study takes a mile-high view of a relatively homogenous population, looking for large trends over time. While population-based studies do not apply to each individual patient, knowing that appropriate treatment of ADHD may prevent criminal behavior is very encouraging. The data for more severe consequences of ADHD in females are particularly interesting, though they may stem from underrecognized mild ADHD in girls.

PRACTICE IMPLICATIONS:

Consider including data about these general trends regarding criminal behavior when discussing risks and benefits of treating ADHD with patients and their caregivers.

Clozapine for Conduct Disorder in Schizophrenia

REVIEW OF: Krakowski M, Tural U, Czobor P. The importance of conduct disorder in the treatment of violence in schizophrenia: Efficacy of clozapine compared with olanzapine and haloperidol. *Am J Psychiatry*. 2021;178(3):266–274. [Published correction appears in *Am J Psychiatry* 2021;178(7):671]

STUDY TYPE: Randomized controlled trial

We often struggle to find effective interventions for aggressive behavior in patients with schizophrenia. For patients with a history of conduct disorder (CD), the task is even more challenging. In a previous study, the authors demonstrated that clozapine is effective in reducing aggression and impulsive behavior in patients with schizophrenia (Krakowski MI et al, *Arch Gen Psychiatry* 2006;63(6):622–629). But will clozapine also reduce aggression in patients who additionally have a history of CD?

The authors examined this question by enrolling 99 subjects with schizophrenia in a 12-week, double-blind trial conducted in a psychiatric research unit. All subjects had a history of being physically assaultive, and about half (n=53) had a history of CD prior to age 15. Subjects were randomly assigned to receive clozapine (n=33), olanzapine (n=34), or haloperidol (n=22), and the frequency and severity of assaults were scored on the Modified Overt Aggression Scale (MOAS). The MOAS total score and the physical assault subscore were compared across groups.

RESULTS:

For all subjects, clozapine was superior to olanzapine and haloperidol in preventing violent behavior, and olanzapine was superior to haloperidol. For subjects with a history of CD, clozapine's efficacy in preventing violence was particularly high: These subjects were over three times as likely to have a lower MOAS score and four times as likely to have a lower physical assault score, compared to subjects on haloperidol. Subjects without CD were 1.9 times as likely to have a lower MOAS score and 2.7 times as likely to have a lower physical assault score with clozapine, compared to subjects on haloperidol.

CARLAT TAKE:

Patients with schizophrenia often show symptoms of CD before age 15, although it may require some digging to establish the diagnosis, since the psychotic disorder may overshadow other symptoms. Although this study's sample size was on the smaller side, clozapine was superior to olanzapine and haloperidol for preventing violent behavior, especially for those with a history of CD.

PRACTICE IMPLICATIONS:

We probably underprescribe clozapine generally, and it's something you should have in your toolbox for patients with schizophrenia and physical aggression or CD.

DASH Diet for Childhood ADHD

REVIEW OF: Khoshbakht Y, Moghtaderi F, Bidaki R, Hosseinzadeh M, Salehi-Abargouei A. The effect of dietary approaches to stop hypertension (DASH) diet on attention-deficit hyperactivity disorder (ADHD) symptoms: A randomized controlled clinical trial. *Eur J Nutr.* 2021;60(7):3647–3658.

STUDY TYPE: Randomized controlled trial

Dietary approaches for controlling ADHD in children have been studied over many decades, but none have been found to be clearly effective. In a recent study, researchers examined the Dietary Approaches to Stop Hypertension (DASH) diet, which includes several interventions that could be helpful in ADHD: more fruit/vegetable intake, higher essential fatty acids from fish, and foods rich in vitamin C, calcium, and magnesium. The DASH diet also limits the intake of simple sugars, artificial sweeteners, and food additives that have been hypothesized to worsen ADHD symptoms.

This randomized controlled trial recruited 80 children with ADHD, ages 6–12 years, to receive the DASH diet or a control diet for 12 weeks. All the children but one were male, and none had ever used medications or behavioral therapy for ADHD. The control diet was meant to resemble a child's typical diet and allowed for more refined grains, full-fat dairy products, and simple sugars. All the diets were designed by nutritionists, who took into account individual caloric and nutritional needs. The children and parents were visited monthly over the study period and completed ADHD assessments and food logs. The severity of ADHD symptoms was measured with various standardized scales, including the Abbreviated Conners Scale.

RESULTS:

At the end of 12 weeks, the children on the DASH diet had significantly greater improvements than control subjects on most scales, including both parent and teacher versions. For example, on the Abbreviated Conners Scale (a 30-point scale), the parent version improved by 4.7 points for the DASH diet group vs 3 points for the intervention group ($p=0.04$), while the teacher version improved more impressively—5.3 points for the DASH diet vs 1.9 for the control ($p<0.001$).

A main limitation of this study was that since researchers cannot ethically recommend unhealthy diets for children, the study's control diet may have been significantly better than what the children were eating before. It's also not clear how generalizable monthly meetings with nutritionists might be. Moreover, this study included only one girl, and all the participants were naïve to any medication or behavioral therapy interventions, calling into question generalizability.

CARLAT TAKE:
While the DASH diet produced results in this study, generalizability may be limited, and pharmacotherapy is still the first-line recommendation for children over 5.

PRACTICE IMPLICATIONS:
The DASH diet for ADHD might be a good place to start for highly motivated parents who wish to avoid medications. For more information on the DASH diet, see www.dashdiet.org.

The Effect of Age and Pubertal Stage on Mental Health in Gender-Incongruent Youth

REVIEW OF: Sorbara JC, Chiniara LN, Thompson S, Palmert MR. Mental health and timing of gender-affirming care. *Pediatrics*. 2020;146(4):e20193600.

STUDY TYPE: Observational study

GENDER INCONGRUENCE MEANS identification with a gender different from the one assigned at birth; youth with gender incongruence have an elevated risk of suicide and other psychiatric problems. Gender-affirming medical care (GAMC), such as hormonal therapies, can reduce those risks, but when is it best to start those treatments?

An earlier study found that psychiatric outcomes were better when youth began GAMC before age 12, compared to those who transitioned in adolescence. This study built on the earlier finding by examining the associations between age and pubertal stage at presentation for GAMC, and mental health.

The researchers undertook a chart review of 300 patients at a Canadian clinic for transgender youth. They compared outcomes for two groups: those presenting before age 15 (n=116, median age 14) and those presenting after age 15 (n=184, median age 16). Most were assigned female at birth (75%), and the majority were White (72%). The rate of autism (6%) was higher than that of the general population, which is a common finding in this population.

RESULTS:

Those who started treatment after age 15 had higher rates of depression (46% vs 30%), self-harm (40% vs 28%), suicide attempts (17% vs 9%), and psychiatric medication use (36% vs 23%). They also recognized their gender incongruence later (median age 9 vs 6) and socially transitioned later (15 vs 13).

Stage of puberty at the time of starting hormones was even more predictive of problems than age. Late pubertal youth (Tanner Stage 4 or 5) were four to five times more likely to report depressive or anxiety disorders. The gender assigned at birth was also predictive, with those transitioning from female to male reporting a three-fold higher rate of self-harm than those transitioning from male to female. Older teens were more likely to be taking psychotropic medications.

The study's main limitation was its uncontrolled design, which left open the possibility that the youth who presented later were already at risk for psychiatric problems. It may be that youth with more secure identities and supportive families are simply more likely to seek these services at a younger age. Further observational research has found that receiving GAMC in adolescence vs adulthood is associated with less suicidal ideation (Turban JL et al, *PLOS ONE* 2022;17(1):e0261039).

CARLAT TAKE:

We have a lot to learn about possible differences between patients who experience gender dysphoria prepubertally vs postpubertally. Still, this study may be reassuring for families who are considering gender-affirming hormones before the onset of puberty. Outcomes are apparently better when treatment is started before secondary sexual characteristics begin to develop.

PRACTICE IMPLICATIONS:

Implications for our current cultural discussion of transgender youth aside, assessing for gender incongruence and GAMC requires a nuanced conversation. The results of this study should be shared with patients and their families.

Electroconvulsive Therapy in Adolescents and Transitional-Age Youth

REVIEW OF: Luccarelli J, McCoy TH, Uchida M, Green A, Seiner SJ, Henry ME. The efficacy and cognitive effects of acute course electroconvulsive therapy are equal in adolescents, transitional age youth, and young adults. *J Child Adolesc Psychopharmacol.* 2021;31(8):538–544.

STUDY TYPE: Retrospective cohort study

Electroconvulsive therapy (ECT) is the most effective treatment available for major depression for adults, with remission rates in the range of 70%–90%. But cognitive side effects have limited the use of ECT to those with treatment-resistant depression. ECT is rarely used for adolescents or young adults; this study adds to our knowledge about the efficacy and safety of ECT in a younger population.

This retrospective study included 424 patients ages 16–30 years who received ECT at a single medical center. Adolescents ages 16 and 17 made up 5.4% of the group, while 62% of the group were transitional-age youth from 18 to 25. About 64% had major depressive disorder. Other diagnoses included bipolar disorder, schizophrenia, schizoaffective disorder, and catatonia. All patients received ECT three times per week, and 95.5% had right unilateral electrode placement. Patients completed assessments for depression (the Quick Inventory of Depressive Symptomatology-Self Report [QIDS]), overall mental health (the Behavior and Symptom Identification Scale-24 [BASIS-24]), and cognition (the Montreal Cognitive Assessment [MoCA]) before and after the first, fifth, and 10th treatments.

RESULTS:

After 10 treatments, the mean QIDS score dropped from 17.0 (±4.9), which is in the range of severe depression, to 10.3 (±5.4), or mild to moderate depression. Adolescents and transitional-age youth showed similar benefits. There was a small average reduction in the MoCA score (-1.1); however, testing occurred 48 hours after ECT, and ECT neurocognitive effects typically improve two to three days after treatments. The drop in cognitive scores was less than what is considered a clinically important difference used in studies of adult stroke patients.

CARLAT TAKE:

While the effect of ECT is less impressive than for adults, this study showed reassuringly little impact on cognitive function in adolescents, transitional-age youth, and young adults. In addition, a recent systematic review revealed that ECT response rates for children and adolescents with unipolar depression ranged from 53% to 77% across various studies (Castaneda-Ramirez S et al, *Eur Child Adolesc Psychiatry.* Published online January 9, 2022).

PRACTICE IMPLICATIONS:

Keep ECT in mind for your adolescent and transitional-age patients with severe treatment-resistant depression.

The Evidence for Polypharmacy in ADHD

REVIEW OF: Baker M, Huefner JC, Bellonci C, Hilt R, Carlson GA. Polypharmacy in the management of attention-deficit/hyperactivity disorder in children and adolescents: A review and update. *J Child Adolesc Psychopharmacol.* 2021;31(3):148–163.

STUDY TYPE: Literature review

Polypharmacy is always a question of additional benefits vs additional side effects. This review examined the evidence for polypharmacy in the treatment of children and adolescents with ADHD, including ADHD with various comorbidities.

The authors' literature search turned up 39 studies, including 17 randomized controlled trials (RCTs), which they characterized as a "relatively limited evidence base . . . to support a practice that occurred in 20% of outpatient visits in 2007 and is likely higher today." Nearly all trials involved stimulants; the most common polypharmacy involved alpha-agonists (16 studies), followed by risperidone and atomoxetine.

RESULTS:

For partial responders to a stimulant for ADHD, the addition of an alpha-agonist was superior to alpha-agonists or stimulants alone, but the combination was associated with bradycardia, sedation, somnolence, and hypotension.

One RCT of atomoxetine found no evidence of improvement with added methylphenidate, and the authors concluded that "optimizing dose and allowing adequate duration for response is favorable to adding medications."

For ADHD with comorbid aggression and disruptive behavior, stimulants alone have a large effect size. Combination treatment with divalproex or risperidone did improve response, with the greatest support for risperidone; however, despite the low dosages of risperidone (<2 mg/day) over short study durations, significant prolactin elevations and weight gain were noted.

For the management of comorbid anxiety, depression, and disruptive mood dysregulation disorder, data from four RCTs of SSRIs with stimulants showed that this common combination, while safe, conveyed minimal benefits for anxiety and mood.

Overall, the authors supported starting with stimulant monotherapy for kids with ADHD. They recommended using measurement-based care to determine if the benefit of an added medication is worth the risk.

CARLAT TAKE:

For stimulants and alpha-agonists, look out for typical alpha-agonist side effects. Considering adding methylphenidate to Strattera? You might be better off switching. For stimulants and risperidone, look out for prolactinemia and weight gain (keeping in mind that pubertal status may play a role in the former). For mood or anxiety problems in the setting of ADHD treated with a stimulant, adding an SSRI is likely to be low yield.

PRACTICE IMPLICATIONS:

Combination treatment for ADHD may be beneficial, though it (unsurprisingly) often makes side effects more likely. This collection of results makes a nice reference for our risk/benefit conversations.

Intravenous Ketamine for Teen Depression

REVIEW OF: Dwyer JB, Landeros-Weisenberger A, Johnson JA, et al. Efficacy of intravenous ketamine in adolescent treatment-resistant depression: A randomized midazolam-controlled trial. *Am J Psychiatry*. 2021;178(4):352–362.

STUDY TYPE: Randomized controlled trial

Treatment-resistant depression (TRD) of teenagers is a growing concern. Although intravenous ketamine is associated with clear and immediate improvement of TRD in adults, there is little research to show its effectiveness in teens. A recent study tried to fill this knowledge gap.

This study was conducted at the Yale Child Study Center. Researchers enrolled 17 teenagers ages 13–17 years with severe major depressive disorder but without active suicidal ideation or comorbid substance use disorder. Teens could continue current psychotropic medications while enrolled. While the participants were required to have failed only one antidepressant trial, on average they had failed three antidepressants and six total psychotropic medications, excluding ADHD medications.

The researchers conducted a randomized, double-blind, active-controlled, crossover study. Patients were given a single infusion of ketamine (0.5 mg/kg) or midazolam (0.045 mg/kg) and switched to the other treatment after two weeks. The primary endpoint was a greater than 50% improvement in the Montgomery-Åsberg Depression Rating Scale (MADRS) score 24 hours after treatment.

RESULTS:

Subjects who received ketamine reported a remarkable improvement in depression following ketamine treatment. Their average baseline MADRS score of 33 dropped significantly lower with ketamine (to 15.4) compared to midazolam (24.1), with a strong effect size of 0.78 (p=0.03). Overall, 75% of the group responded to ketamine, compared to 35% with midazolam. Two weeks following the infusion, responders to ketamine maintained partial improvement in depression, whereas responders to midazolam returned to their baseline level of depression. The main adverse effects seen with ketamine were an increase in pulse and blood pressure during the infusion—as well as dissociation up to two hours after the infusion.

CARLAT TAKE:
Ketamine worked well for the teens in this study, but given the dissociation some of them experienced, future research might investigate a lower dosing protocol. As with ketamine for adults, how long to continue treatment remains unclear. Future research should also include teens with suicidal ideation.

PRACTICE IMPLICATIONS:
This study supports ketamine as an option for teens with TRD. Given the lack of data on how long-term use affects the adolescent brain, it's probably best used when other options have failed.

Long-Term Treatment Response in Pediatric OCD

REVIEW OF: Melin K, Skarphedinsson G, Thomsen PH, et al. Treatment gains are sustainable in pediatric obsessive-compulsive disorder: Three-year follow-up from the NordLOTS. *J Am Acad Child Adolesc Psychiatry*. 2020;59(2):244–253.

STUDY TYPE: Randomized controlled trial

OCD affects 1%–4% of children and adolescents and can be chronically debilitating in 40%–60% of cases. The 2004 Pediatric OCD Treatment Study (POTS) showed that cognitive behavioral therapy (CBT) and sertraline had comparable benefits over 12 weeks of treatment. However, OCD is a chronic condition, and treatment options in the long run are less clear. For example, when youths do not respond to CBT within 12–16 sessions, should we continue CBT or recommend pharmacotherapy? The current study addressed that question.

The Nordic Long-Term OCD Treatment Study (NordLOTS) enrolled 269 children and adolescents (ages 7–17 years) with OCD from clinics across Sweden, Norway, and Denmark. Children's Yale-Brown Obsessive-Compulsive Scale (CY-BOCS) scores were used as inclusion criteria (>15) and to deem subjects as responders (0–15), nonresponders (16–40), or in remission (0–10).

All participants were treated with 14 weeks of manualized, exposure-based CBT. Nonresponders to weekly CBT (n=64) were randomized to continue CBT (n=28) for 10 more sessions or switch to sertraline (n=26) titrated at 25–200 mg over 16 weeks. Subjects were followed periodically for three years.

RESULTS:

About 65% of all participants responded to initial CBT, and these responders maintained their treatment effect with a significant decrease in their CY-BOCS total scores at one-year follow-up.

Nonresponders to initial CBT had significantly more severe OCD at baseline (CY-BOCS 26.4 vs 23.8; p<0.001). Surprisingly, they did equally well with continued CBT vs switching to sertraline (p=0.169), and caught up with responders at three-year follow-up (CY-BOCS=5.0 for both). At three years, 73% (n=196) of the total sample were in remission, with 24% having CY-BOCS scores of 0. Of the remainder, 17% (n=46) had mild symptoms (CY-BOCS=11.0–15.0); 10% (n=27) had moderate or severe symptoms (CY-BOCS≥16.0).

CARLAT TAKE:

Manualized exposure-based CBT remains an excellent approach for pediatric OCD, but for some kids, we need to continue treatment beyond 14 weeks. In contrast to adult studies showing that CBT benefits may endure better than medication treatment once treatment ends (Ponniah K et al, *J Obsessive Compuls Relat Disord* 2013;2(2):207–218), this study showed that at three years, SSRIs are just as effective for children who fail or are unable to access CBT.

PRACTICE IMPLICATIONS:

With CBT and/or sertraline, if longer-term care is available, the prognosis for pediatric OCD is good.

New Canadian Guidelines for Eating Disorders in Children

REVIEW OF: Couturier J, Isserlin L, Norris M, et al. Canadian practice guidelines for the treatment of children and adolescents with eating disorders. *J Eat Disord*. 2020;8:4.

STUDY TYPE: Systematic review

In 2020, a 24-member team of Canadian psychiatrists, parents, and patient representatives published new practice guidelines for eating disorders. Their systematic review screened thousands of abstracts to find several dozen articles, prioritizing randomized controlled trials. They assessed psychotherapies, including family-based therapy, cognitive behavioral therapy (CBT), and dialectical behavior therapy; medications (primarily atypical antipsychotics and SSRIs); and treatment sites.

Of the studies reviewed, many suffered from significant potential bias, and many showed no significant effect of treatment. There were some interesting positive studies; one compared CBT with psychodynamic therapy for 81 girls with anorexia nervosa. The two treatments were comparable, each yielding remission rates of about 33% after an average of 37 weeks of treatment.

RESULTS:

After synthesizing the studies, the researchers arrived at two main recommendations. First, family-based treatment is clearly effective for both anorexia nervosa and bulimia nervosa. Second, less restrictive treatment environments (eg, family-based or day treatments) are more effective than lengthy hospitalizations. The following five modalities were also recommended, but with less confidence: multifamily therapy, CBT, adolescent-focused psychotherapy, yoga, and olanzapine or aripiprazole with anorexia nervosa "if monitored carefully."

CARLAT TAKE:
Eating disorders in children and adolescents are not easily treated pharmacologically, which makes them harder to study and complicates the establishment of definite treatment algorithms even after a concerted approach by a multidisciplinary team. However, less-restrictive treatments, and family-based treatments, are preferable.

PRACTICE IMPLICATIONS:
This exhaustive review favors evidence-based psychotherapies, particularly family-based treatments, in the least restrictive environments for children and adolescents suffering from eating disorders.

A Novel Treatment for Dramatic-Onset Autoimmune OCD or Severe Food Restriction?

REVIEW OF: Melamed I, Kobayashi RH, O'Connor M, et al. Evaluation of intravenous immunoglobulin in pediatric acute-onset neuropsychiatric syndrome. *J Child Adolesc Psychopharmacol.* 2021;31(2):118–128.

STUDY TYPE: Open-label trial

Pediatric acute-onset neuropsychiatric syndrome (PANS) is defined by the dramatic, abrupt onset of obsessions, compulsions, and/or eating restrictions along with two neuropsychiatric symptoms, most commonly tics, anxiety disorders, urinary difficulties, and oppositional behavior. The pathophysiology of PANS is not known, but it is suspected in some cases to have an autoimmune etiology and is therefore sometimes treated with intravenous immunoglobulin (IVIG); psychiatric medications and antibiotics have also been used. This industry-funded study tested an extended IVIG dosing strategy.

Twenty-one patients, ages 4–16 years, with moderate to severe PANS symptoms on the Pediatric Acute Neuropsychiatric Symptom Scale, were recruited from seven sites. Most were male (62%) with a mean duration of PANS symptoms of 4.3 years. Participants remained on any antibiotics they'd been taking if doses were stable for the prior three months. They received six IVIG infusions dosed at 1 g/kg and given every three weeks.

Primary outcome measures included the Children's Yale-Brown Obsessive-Compulsive Scale (CY-BOCS) and Clinical Global Impressions Scale (CGI-S), measured at baseline and repeated at one and eight weeks after the final infusion. The Parent-Rated PANS Questionnaire (PRPQ), developed for this study, captured interim efficacy data at each infusion. A subset of patients participated in a 46-week follow-up visit. Patient diaries tracked adverse events.

RESULTS:

The IVIG infusions were effective. All primary outcome measures decreased significantly. CY-BOCS fell by 61.45% (p<0.0002), CGI-S by 44% (p<0.0001), and Yale Global Tic Severity Scale (YGTSS) by 66.61% (p=0.0005). The PRPQ did not show improvement until the third infusion but dropped 52.82% (p=0.004) from baseline to the last infusion.

At 46-week follow-up, most of the improvements persisted except for tics; however, tic severity remained below baseline measures. The treatment was well tolerated; side effects were transient and mild and included post-infusion headache, nausea, and vomiting.

CARLAT TAKE:
While the results are promising, this was a small, uncontrolled, open-label trial, and the lack of a control group precludes measuring an effect size.

PRACTICE IMPLICATIONS:
This was an important proof-of-concept trial of IVIG for moderate to severe PANS.

SSRIs and Hydroxyzine for Avoidant/Restrictive Food Intake Disorder?

REVIEW OF: Mahr F, Billman M, Essayli JH, Lane Loney SE. Selective serotonin reuptake inhibitors and hydroxyzine in the treatment of avoidant/restrictive food intake disorder in children and adolescents: Rationale and evidence. *J Child Adolesc Psychopharmacol.* 2022;32(2):117–121.

STUDY TYPE: Retrospective chart review

Clinicians use olanzapine, mirtazapine, and other appetite-inducing medications off label to treat avoidant/restrictive food intake disorder (ARFID), but with little research to support their use. This study unpacked the potential role of medications in treating comorbid symptoms associated with ARFID.

Researchers reviewed the charts of 53 children and teens with ARFID treated in a partial hospital program. The group was largely pubertal females with body mass index (BMI) of about 15–16. All had significant anxiety. These charts were selected because the patients were given SSRIs alone or with hydroxyzine as part of their treatment. Those who took hydroxyzine in addition to SSRIs were older than those who did not (13 vs 11), were 64% female vs 92%, and had more depressive symptoms on the Child Depression Inventory (62 vs 53). This study followed the percent median body mass index (%MBMI, ie, the patient's BMI/the median BMI for age x 100) to track progress with weight gain. A typical goal is for patients to achieve a %MBMI of 90 to consider the treatment clinically meaningful.

RESULTS:

All patients benefited from SSRIs, with reduced anxiety, depression, and fear of eating. Patients in both categories gained weight, with those on SSRIs alone experiencing a %MBMI increase from 88 to 96 over the course of a year, and those who received SSRI + hydroxyzine up from 89 to 98 over the same period. Hydroxyzine also helped subjective fear of eating as well as nausea in the more severe cohort of patients who received both medications. Side effects included mild sedation and fatigue for hydroxyzine, and headache for SSRIs.

The authors suggested starting SSRIs at 5 mg of fluoxetine (or equivalent) and titrating slowly to prevent paradoxically increasing anxiety. Hydroxyzine takes 15–30 minutes to act and peaks around two hours. They recommended dosing 0.5 mg/kg every four to six hours as needed for anxiety. (Fluoxetine and hydroxyzine liquid can be helpful for patients who have trouble swallowing pills.)

CARLAT TAKE:
While this was a small uncontrolled study of patients in a relatively high level of care, it reminds us to assess anxiety and depression when treating ARFID. More severe symptoms benefited from more medication, but as expected, the increase in medication was associated with more side effects.

PRACTICE IMPLICATIONS:

We need more research, but in the meantime, SSRIs may help with anxiety and weight gain for children and teens suffering from ARFID; adding hydroxyzine to an SSRI may help with more severe symptoms.

Viloxazine for ADHD in Children and Adolescents

REVIEW OF: Nasser A, Kosheleff AR, Hull JT, et al. Evaluating the likelihood to be helped or harmed after treatment with viloxazine extended-release in children and adolescents with attention-deficit/hyperactivity disorder. *Int J Clin Pract*. 2021;75(8):e14330.

STUDY TYPE: Post-hoc analysis of randomized controlled trials

In 2021, viloxazine (Qelbree) received FDA approval for the treatment of ADHD in children and adolescents (in 2022, after this research update was originally published, Qelbree was also approved for adults). Like atomoxetine (Strattera), viloxazine is an SNRI that has been used as an antidepressant in Europe. For ADHD, stimulants are still the most effective medications, but how does this new non-stimulant option measure up?

RESULTS:

The analysis included four randomized controlled trials (RCTs), all double-blind. When analyzed together, they showed viloxazine was more effective than placebo at reducing ADHD symptoms in a combined 1,354 children and adolescents. On an individual level, three of the four trials were positive. All four trials used improvement in the ADHD Rating Scale (ADHD-RS) after five weeks of treatment as their primary outcome. There were two levels of improvement: a 30% improvement, and a more clinically significant 50% improvement, in ADHD-RS scores.

The authors converted these results into more relevant figures: number needed to treat (NNT) and number needed to harm (NNH). (See "A Quick Primer on Assessing Scientific Research" at the beginning of this book; in this case, "harm" was defined as discontinuing the trial due to any adverse effect.) For these studies, the NNT was 6 (95% CI [5, 9]) for the less stringent 30% improvement in ADHD-RS and 7 (95% CI [5, 10]) for the 50% improvement level. The NNH was 46 (95% CI [26, 167]), meaning one in 46 patients discontinued the medication due to side effects for both 30% and 50% levels of improvement. The most common side effects were somnolence, decreased appetite, and headache. By contrast, other analyses have found similar NNTs for atomoxetine (5–7) and better NNTs for traditional stimulants (2–4).

Two main weaknesses stand out. The analysis was industry sponsored, as were the four RCTs it analyzed. However, a 2022 meta-analysis of viloxazine for child/adolescent ADHD included all of these studies, plus one other; it assessed the studies as having a low risk of bias, and concluded that viloxazine was significantly better than placebo (Singh A et al, *J Cent Nerv Syst Dis* 2022;14:11795735221092522). The other weakness in the data is generalizability—other significant mental or neurological disorders were exclusion criteria for the four studies.

CHILD AND ADOLESCENT PSYCHIATRY

CARLAT TAKE:
In children and adolescents with ADHD, viloxazine is reportedly well tolerated with an efficacy comparable to atomoxetine but less than that of the stimulants.

PRACTICE IMPLICATIONS:
For kids and teens with ADHD who are not good candidates for a stimulant and are able to afford a brand-name drug, viloxazine is now an option.

Vitamin D for ADHD?

REVIEW OF: Gan J, Galer P, Ma D, Chen C, Xiong T. The effect of vitamin D supplementation on attention-deficit/hyperactivity disorder: A systematic review and meta-analysis of randomized controlled trials. *J Child Adolesc Psychopharmacol.* 2019;29(9):670–687.

STUDY TYPE: Systematic review and meta-analysis

MANY CHILDREN DO not respond to or tolerate standard pharmacotherapies, driving continued interest in supplements for many conditions, including ADHD. Vitamin D plays a role in healthy brain development, and vitamin D deficiency causes neurotransmitter alterations in pathways associated with ADHD. But is there a link between ADHD and lower vitamin D levels? These researchers conducted a systematic review and meta-analysis to assess the evidence to date.

The study looked at four randomized controlled trials (RCTs) studying vitamin D supplementation for ADHD (1,000 units daily to 50,000 units weekly) versus placebo as adjuncts to methylphenidate for children 5–18 years old (n=256). Trials lasted six to 12 weeks. Their primary outcome was ADHD severity, based on a variety of parent-only rating scales. Secondary outcomes were adverse effects of supplementation and vitamin D status afterward.

RESULTS:

Adjunctive vitamin D supplementation yielded a small but statistically significant improvement in ADHD total score and in subscales for inattention, hyperactivity, and behavior. Scores for oppositional behaviors were unchanged, except in a subgroup analysis of high-dose vitamin D supplementation (>2,000 international units [IUs] daily). Notably, one study found that children with baseline vitamin D deficiency or insufficiency were more likely to respond to adjunctive vitamin D supplementation. Only one trial reported adverse effects. These were mild and similar between groups. Not surprisingly, vitamin D supplementation increased vitamin D levels and increased the ratio of patients with sufficient vitamin D levels.

This paper used excellent methodological procedures for conducting systematic reviews and meta-analyses. Unfortunately, the RCTs were of low or very low quality. Randomization procedures were not clear, the total population was less than 400, and statistical methods varied. All of these trials were carried out in the Middle East, but the ethnicities of participants were not reported, so generalizability is not clear.

CARLAT TAKE:
Vitamin D supplementation is a relatively low-risk and low-cost intervention with other potential health benefits. It's unclear whether similar results would extend to non-methylphenidate stimulants. More research is also needed to examine whether vitamin D dose, administration frequency, and baseline vitamin D levels influence outcomes.

PRACTICE IMPLICATIONS:

Consider vitamin D supplementation for children with ADHD, especially alongside vitamin D deficiency, in combination with standard ADHD treatment. Take care to avoid megadoses, which can disrupt calcium metabolism or result in toxicity. See "Recommended Vitamin D Dose" table below.

TABLE: Recommended Vitamin D Dose

Age (years)	Daily Requirement (IU)	Upper-Level Daily Intake (IU)
0–1	400	1000
1–9	400	2000
11–18	400	4000

Source: EFSA and ESPGHAN (www.academic.oup.com/jcem/article/99/4/1132/2537181)

Which Medications Have the Lowest Risk of Side Effects?

REVIEW OF: Solmi M, Fornaro M, Ostinelli EG, et al. Safety of 80 antidepressants, antipsychotics, anti-attention-deficit/hyperactivity medications and mood stabilizers in children and adolescents with psychiatric disorders: A large scale systematic meta-review of 78 adverse effects. *World Psychiatry*. 2020;19(2):214–232.

STUDY TYPE: Systematic review and meta-analysis

ADVERSE EFFECTS ARE important considerations when choosing psychotropic medications, especially in children and adolescents. This study pooled available research to compare the safety profiles of various psychotropics used in the pediatric population. After screening thousands of studies for 78 possible adverse effects, the authors analyzed data from nine network meta-analyses, 39 meta-analyses, 90 randomized controlled trials, and eight cohort studies. The combined sample of these studies included 337,686 children and adolescents: 120,000 on antidepressants, 66,000 on antipsychotics, 148,000 on ADHD meds, and 1,600 on mood stabilizers.

RESULTS:

Among antidepressants, escitalopram and fluoxetine fared best, while venlafaxine was worst owing to reports of anorexia, abdominal pain, hypertension, and suicidality. Sertraline also performed poorly due to gastrointestinal issues, insomnia, and weight gain. Among antipsychotics, lurasidone was found to be the least problematic, with asenapine in second place. Olanzapine was the most problematic, carrying a host of side effects including sedation, metabolic syndrome, and extrapyramidal side effects, with aripiprazole in second-to-last place.

Turning to ADHD medications, methylphenidate stood out as safest, although only slightly ahead of lisdexamfetamine, while atomoxetine was the worst of the lot due to gastrointestinal issues and weight loss. Surprisingly, guanfacine also had significant issues, such as reports of abdominal pain, sedation, and, notably, QT prolongation.

Finally, among the mood stabilizers, lithium was the most tolerated, while valproate trailed the pack with significant adverse effects like weight gain, sedation, and cytopenia.

CARLAT TAKE:

This study yielded some surprising results and is worth a close read. While venlafaxine's higher side effect profile was expected, we had not imagined sertraline to do so much worse than escitalopram and fluoxetine. Furthermore, we had, perhaps incorrectly, considered guanfacine and atomoxetine mild "starter" medications, even placebo-like, but here the stimulants stood out for their advantages in both safety and efficacy. Lastly, lithium and lurasidone may deserve stronger consideration, despite having bloodwork and insurance issues respectively.

PRACTICE IMPLICATIONS:
The agents with the fewest side effects are escitalopram and fluoxetine for depression, lurasidone for schizophrenia, methylphenidate for ADHD, and lithium for bipolar disorder.

GERIATRIC PSYCHIATRY

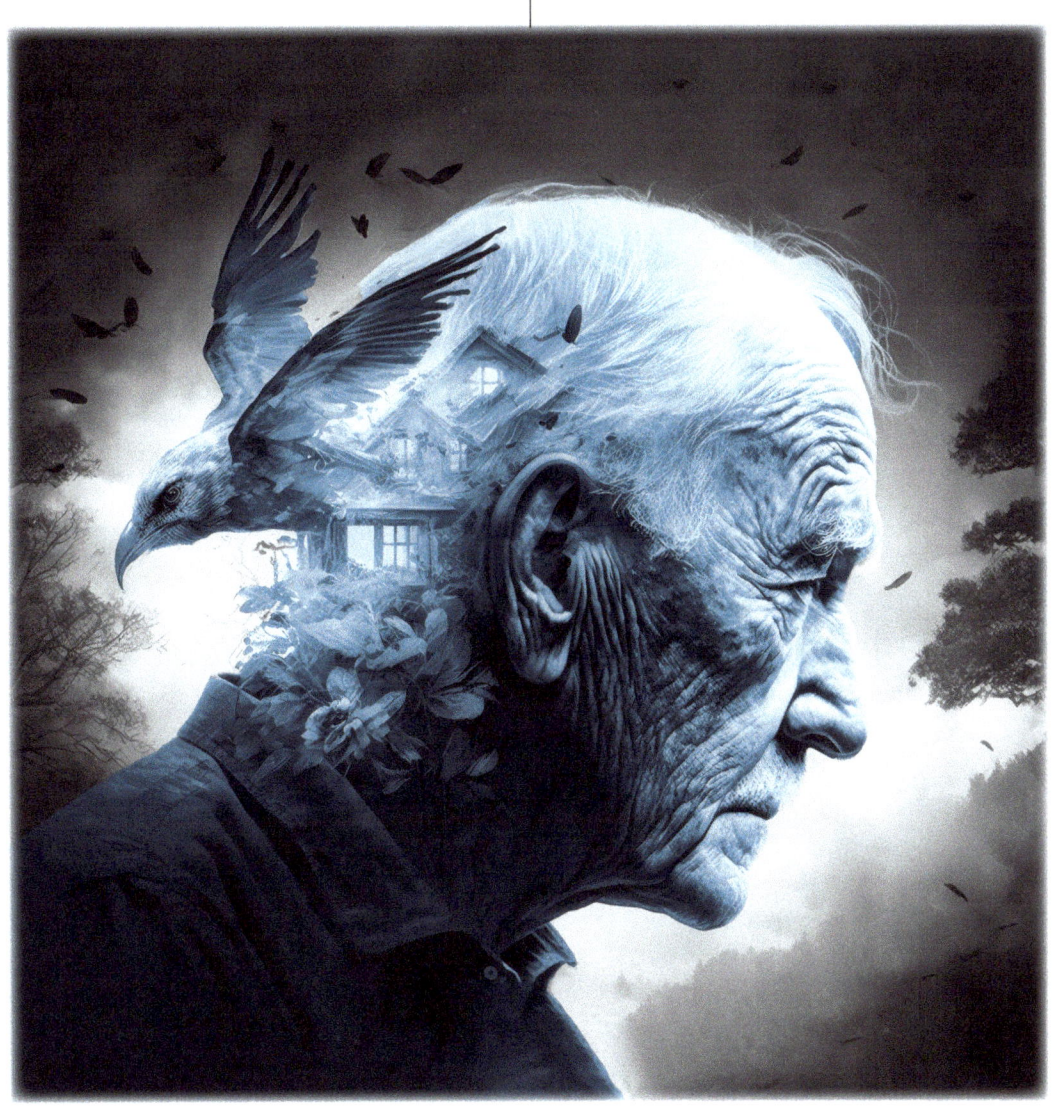

Does Mirtazapine Treat Agitation in Dementia?

REVIEW OF: Banerjee S, High J, Stirling S, et al. Study of mirtazapine for agitated behaviours in dementia (SYMBAD): A randomised, double-blind, placebo-controlled trial. *Lancet.* 2021;398(10310):1487–1497.

STUDY TYPE: Randomized controlled trial

AGITATION OFTEN ACCOMPANIES dementia. While behavioral interventions are first line, they are often not fully effective. A variety of medications can be used to treat behavioral symptoms, but not without risk. Antipsychotics increase mortality rates in patients with dementia. SSRIs such as citalopram are safer and have some efficacy, but what about mirtazapine? The Study of Mirtazapine for Agitated Behaviors in Dementia (SYMBAD) trial looked at the sedating antidepressant mirtazapine to address agitation associated with Alzheimer's dementia.

This double-blind, placebo-controlled, randomized trial was conducted in 26 UK sites over 12 weeks. It included 204 patients with possible or probable Alzheimer's dementia and with significant agitation as defined by a Cohen-Mansfield Agitation Inventory (CMAI) score of ≥45. 102 patients were randomized to the mirtazapine group (average age 82, 75% female) and 102 patients to the placebo group (average age 82, 58% female). The patients in the mirtazapine group received mirtazapine titrated up to a target dose of 45 mg daily with an average daily dose of 30 mg.

RESULTS:

The primary outcome of change in CMAI did not differ between the two groups. Secondary outcomes included CMAI score at six weeks, quality-of-life measures, cognition and other neuropsychiatric symptoms, and caregiver burden. Only the last was statistically different and showed that caregivers reported more burnout in the mirtazapine group.

Another disappointing result was higher mortality in the mirtazapine group (seven patients) versus the placebo group (one patient). We have little information on the causes of death (a few were coded as "dementia"). As the study was not sufficiently powered to detect mortality differences, and four deaths occurred before week six, these deaths may have happened by chance. Post-hoc analysis showed the difference to be of marginal statistical significance (p=0.065).

One potential limitation of the study was that patients were titrated to a relatively high average dose of mirtazapine—30 mg. This may be too high in the frail elderly and could theoretically cause agitation due to noradrenergic or dopaminergic effects, which may overwhelm sedative effects at high doses. We have few baseline characteristics of the two groups (eg, medical comorbidities), and we would have liked to see certain confounders addressed, including polypharmacy and delirium.

CARLAT TAKE:
Treating agitation associated with Alzheimer's dementia is difficult. So far, no studies of pharmacological interventions have shown consistently positive results.

PRACTICE IMPLICATIONS:
While this study had limitations, it decreases confidence in mirtazapine as a primary anti-agitation treatment in dementia, at least at doses higher than 15 mg. First-line options for behavioral and psychological symptoms of dementia continue to include caregiver education and nonpharmacologic treatments.

Less Sleep Correlated With Dementia

REVIEW OF: Sabia S, Fayosse A, Dumurgier J, et al. Association of sleep duration in middle and old age with incidence of dementia. *Nat Commun.* 2021;12(1):2289.

STUDY TYPE: Prospective cohort study

How is sleep related to dementia? Prior studies among middle-aged and older adults found that both longer and shorter sleep durations are associated with an increased dementia risk. However, as the follow-up duration of those studies was less than 10 years, it is challenging to determine whether sleep irregularities contributed to dementia or reflected its early symptoms.

This study used data from 7,959 participants of the Whitehall II cohort study in the UK to examine the association between sleep duration at ages 50, 60, and 70 and incident dementia over the following 25 years. All patients reported their sleep by questionnaire, and for about 3,900 of them, accelerometer-based data were also available. 521 participants developed dementia over this time period at an average age of 77.

RESULTS:

The researchers found that sleeping less than six hours over the span of ages 50, 60, and 70 was associated with a 30% increased dementia risk compared to those getting normal sleep (defined as seven hours). The study controlled for sociodemographic, behavioral, cardiometabolic, and mental health factors (such as depressive symptoms or central nervous system drugs) that may affect sleep and dementia risk.

The number of long sleepers (eight hours or more) was too small in this study to associate with dementia risk. Additional limitations of this study included the use of electronic medical records to assess dementia cases, which might misclassify milder cases, and incomplete data on the types of dementia.

CARLAT TAKE:

We know there is an association between sleep and cognitive function, likely related to the role of sleep in learning and memory, synaptic plasticity, and waste clearance from the brain. This study supports the association between a short sleep duration in middle life and an increased risk for dementia. This is only a correlation, but a randomized clinical trial assigning patients to poor vs normal sleep and following them for 10–20 years would not be possible.

PRACTICE IMPLICATIONS:

These findings are suggestive and remind us of the primary importance of sleep for sound psychiatric health. Everyone can always benefit from good sleep habits—particularly those at higher risk for dementia.

Listening to Depression: The Importance of Addressing Hearing Loss

REVIEW OF: Marques T, Marques FD, Miguéis A. Age-related hearing loss, depression, and auditory amplification: A randomized clinical trial. *Eur Arch Otorhinolaryngol.* 2022;279(3):1317–1321.

STUDY TYPE: Randomized, open-label, controlled trial

Age-related hearing loss is associated with depression; poorer physical and social functioning; and decreased quality of life, but can hearing aids reverse those trends? This study examined the effects of "aural rehabilitation" (hearing aids) on depressive symptoms.

The study randomly assigned 61 patients with moderate bilateral hearing loss to receive either a hearing aid or a control treatment of follow-up appointments. The treatment group was younger than the control, with an average age of 77 versus 82, a significant difference (p=0.013). The primary outcome was the change in the Geriatric Depression Scale (GDS) at four weeks. A diagnosis of major depression was not required for study entry, but the participants entered the study with an average score on the GDS that was just at the cutoff for depression. Patients with cognitive impairment were excluded from the study.

RESULTS:

After four weeks, the average depression score decreased from 10.63 to 6.94 in the hearing aid group, while the score in the control group went from 11.69 to 10.97, a difference that was significant (p=0.003). Using a regression model, the authors also examined the effect of various factors on depression score: age, marital status, educational level, and ear pure-tone average (a measure of hearing loss). Investigators concluded that hearing loss was independently associated with depression and that the degree of hearing loss was the main predictive factor for depressive symptoms at study entry.

The main limitation of this study was the lack of a placebo treatment in the control arm. Other limitations included the absence of blinding, the brevity of the study, and the disparity in age between the two groups.

CARLAT TAKE:
Many of us have seen dramatic changes in the functionality and demeanor of our elderly patients with restoration of hearing, and it's nice to see that confirmed here, despite the study's limitations.

PRACTICE IMPLICATIONS:
Ask older depressed patients, or others at risk, about hearing loss, and refer to audiology if needed.

Low Vitamin B_{12} Associated With Depression in Older Adults

REVIEW OF: Laird E, O'Halloran AM, Molloy AM, et al. Low vitamin B12 but not folate is associated with incident depressive symptoms in community-dwelling older adults: A 4-year longitudinal study. *Br J Nutr*. 2021;1–8. [Published online ahead of print, 2021 December 13]

STUDY TYPE: Prospective cohort study

Deficiencies of both vitamin B_{12} and folate are highly prevalent among older adults. Depending on the study, 5%–40% of adults older than 50 years have B_{12} deficiency. Folate deficiency ranges from 1.2% among older adults in countries that mandate folate fortification (such as the US) to 31% in countries without this policy (such as the UK). Low concentrations of both B_{12} and folate have been correlated with depression in cross-sectional studies; this recent large longitudinal study adds to the evidence base.

The Irish Longitudinal Study on Aging followed 3,849 people who were all at least 50 years old. At baseline, participants underwent measurements including B_{12} and folate levels, as well as depression screenings with the Center for Epidemiological Studies Depression Scale (CES-D-8). They were reevaluated after two and four years.

RESULTS:

Participants with deficient-low B_{12} status at baseline (<185 pmol/L) had a 51% increased likelihood of developing depression over four years. There was no association between folate status and depression. These findings remained robust after controlling for physical activity, chronic disease burden, vitamin D levels, cardiovascular disease, and antidepressant use.

CARLAT TAKE:

These results point to an association, and no causal relationship can be drawn. Perhaps older depressed patients have poorer appetite or diets. There's also an established correlation between older adults and lower B_{12} levels that may have to do with gastric acidity. Yet whichever way the relationship goes, addressing the possibility of low B_{12}, a water-soluble vitamin, makes sense for older depressed adults.

PRACTICE IMPLICATIONS:

Checking a B_{12} level in depressed older adults is not standard care but may be reasonable. If the level is low, supplementation is a low-cost, relatively safe intervention but may not affect risk of depression.

Rest Easy: Benzos, Z-Drugs, and Dementia

REVIEW OF: Osler M, Jørgensen MB. Associations of benzodiazepines, z-drugs, and other anxiolytics with subsequent dementia in patients with affective disorders: A nationwide cohort and nested case-control study. *Am J Psychiatry*. 2020;177(6):497–505.

STUDY TYPE: Case-control study

Few psychotropics stir controversy like the benzodiazepines. While they work well for anxiety and insomnia, their risks of abuse and dependence have always nagged at us. Some research has suggested that long-term use increases the risk of dementia. (And, as the "z-hypnotics" [eszopiclone, zaleplon, and zolpidem] also act on GABA-A receptors, they have also fallen under suspicion.) Those studies did not control for the underlying diagnosis, and this new study partially overcame that problem by focusing on a homogenous diagnostic group.

This cohort and nested case-control study drew its data from Danish hospital and pharmacy registries. 235,000 patients presented for their first hospitalization for a mood disorder; they were assessed for dementia and followed for three to 11 years. The primary outcome was the difference in the rate of dementia between those who were started on a benzodiazepine or z-hypnotic and those who were not.

Dementia can present with symptoms of depression, so it's possible that some of the patients who converted to dementia were in the early phase of cognitive decline at the start of the study. To control for that, patients who converted to dementia in the first two years were analyzed separately.

The data collected from registries allowed researchers to see all diagnoses, prescribed medications, amounts of medications filled, hospitalizations, timing of diagnoses, and other data prior to study entry. The investigators adjusted for a number of these variables, including gender, age, marital status, education, depression subtype, year of diagnosis, psychotropic medication use, and comorbidity. The thoroughness of their adjustments is what makes this study stand apart in generalizability from prior, similar case-control and prospective studies.

RESULTS:

Of the roughly 235,000 patients included in the study, 4% were diagnosed with dementia. Unexpectedly, there was a decreased risk of dementia in the first two years after study entry if a benzodiazepine or z-drug was prescribed (hazard ratio 0.70, range 0.66–0.74). For years two through 20 after study entry, there was no association between dementia and use of benzodiazepines or z-drugs, even when stratifying based on number of prescriptions, duration of use, combined use, and half-life. A 2021 meta-analysis of 35 studies further undermined the purported link between sedative-hypnotics and dementia, finding no association after controlling for confounders (AlDawsari A et al, *Br J Clin Pharmacol* 2022;88(4):1567–1589).

CARLAT TAKE:
These studies significantly weaken prior findings of an association between benzos/z-hypnotics and dementia.

PRACTICE IMPLICATIONS:
These medications still warrant caution in the elderly due to their risks of falls, oversedation, traffic accidents, and respiratory suppression. Low doses of short-acting benzodiazepines like lorazepam and oxazepam minimize those risks, but nonpharmacological approaches remain first line.

SSRIs and Intracerebral Hemorrhage Risk

REVIEW OF: Kubiszewski P, Sugita L, Kourkoulis C, et al. Association of selective serotonin reuptake inhibitor use after intracerebral hemorrhage with hemorrhage recurrence and depression severity. *JAMA Neurol.* 2020;78(1):1–8.

STUDY TYPE: Prospective cohort study

Depression after strokes is very common, affecting about 50% of all stroke patients. Many such patients are treated with SSRIs, which are generally effective but potentially dangerous, because they can increase the risk of bleeding due to impaired platelet aggregation. This is especially dangerous in intracerebral hemorrhage (ICH), which causes half of all stroke mortality even though it represents only 10%–15% of all strokes. A recent study examined the safety of SSRIs in patients who had recently had an ICH.

This was a longitudinal study in which researchers recruited a total of 1,279 patients (mean age 71.3 years) who were treated for ICH at a single academic hospital from January 2006 to December 2017. Of these patients, 766 were diagnosed with depression, and 281 were started on SSRIs. Patients receiving SSRIs were divided into two categories: high or low risk for a recurrent hemorrhagic stroke. High risk criteria included a history of prior ICH; presence of apolipoprotein *ε2/ε4 gene variants; Black or Hispanic race; and lobar ICH, as opposed to deeper tissues such as the basal ganglia, brainstem, and cerebellum.

RESULTS:

SSRI use was associated with higher ICH recurrence (hazard ratio [HR] 1.3). 6.1% of high-risk patients on SSRIs had a recurrent ICH vs only 3.8% of those not on SSRIs. In contrast, low-risk patients on SSRIs were not at higher risk for a recurrence than those not taking an antidepressant (2.9% vs 2.3%). On the positive side, SSRIs were effective at resolving post-stroke depression, with patients on SSRIs 1.5 times more likely to experience remission. Low doses of SSRIs (<50% max recommended dose) were just as effective as high doses (>50% max recommended dose) and were associated with a lower risk of ICH recurrence (HR 1.25 and 1.61 respectively).

CARLAT TAKE:
High-risk patients are at an increased risk of repeat hemorrhage when SSRIs are used to treat post-ICH depression. This study doesn't address why Black or Hispanic stroke survivors faced higher risk of repeat ICH, but several factors may play a role, including historical undertreatment and injustice.

PRACTICE IMPLICATIONS:
When treating patients for post-ICH stroke depression, discuss the risk of recurrent ICH and consider mirtazapine, bupropion, or half-dose (or lower) SSRIs.

MANAGING ADVERSE EFFECTS

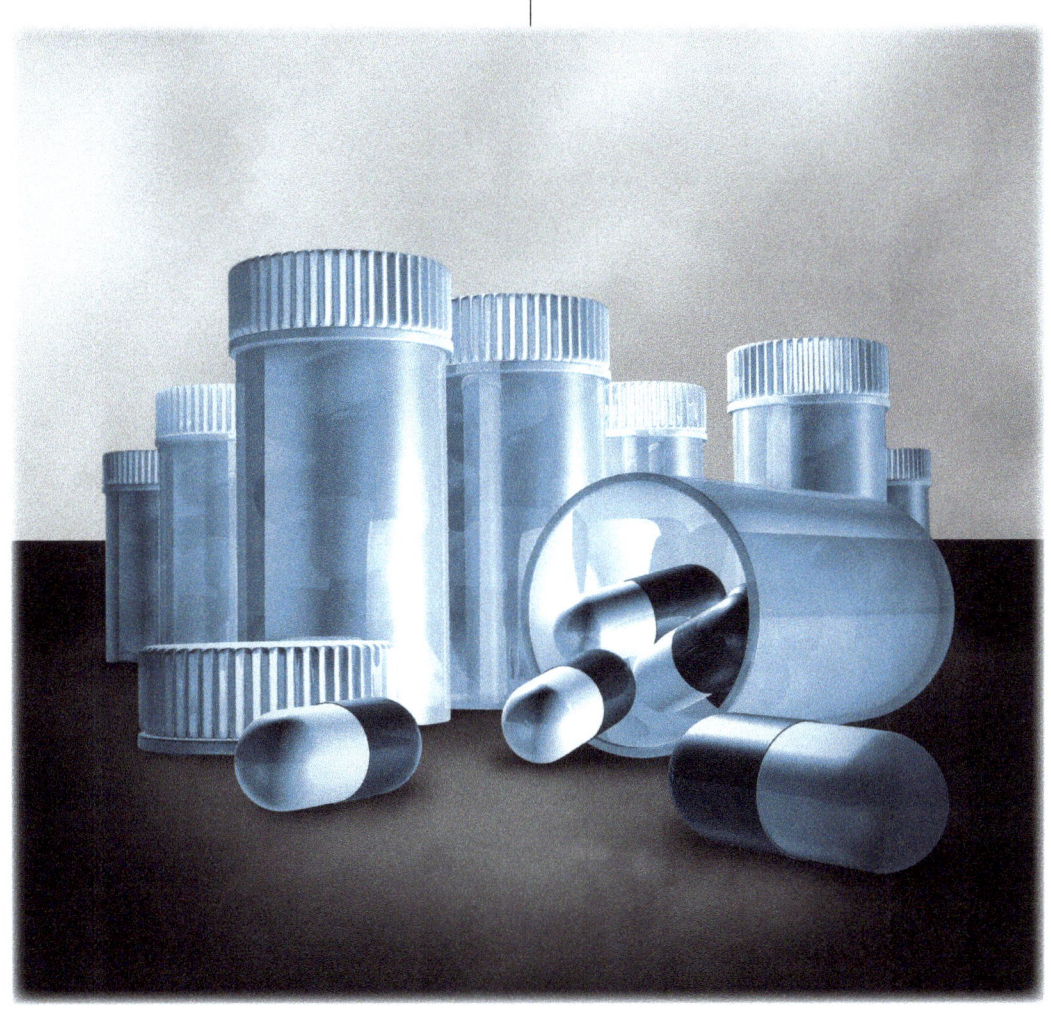

Anticholinergic-Associated Cognitive Impairment in Schizophrenia

REVIEW OF: Joshi YB, Thomas ML, Braff DL, et al. Anticholinergic medication burden-associated cognitive impairment in schizophrenia. *Am J Psychiatry*. 2021;178(9):838–847.

STUDY TYPE: Cross-sectional study

SCHIZOPHRENIA IS ASSOCIATED with impaired cognition. Medications with anticholinergic properties can worsen this problem, including antipsychotics, benztropine, and antidepressants, and may confer an increased risk of dementia. What we don't know is the size of this impact on cognition, which this study investigated.

Researchers examined the magnitude and types of medications with anticholinergic properties. They assessed both global cognition and cognitive subdomains in 1,120 adult outpatients under age 65 with schizophrenia or schizoaffective disorder and enrolled in the larger Consortium on the Genetics of Schizophrenia-2 study. Most were young (mean 24 years); 69% of subjects were male, 43% were White, and 40% were Black. Researchers assessed psychopathology, anticholinergic burden (using the Anticholinergic Cognitive Burden [ACB] scale), and cognition (using the Penn Computerized Neurocognitive Battery). The ACB is a validated expert rating scale that assigns dose-independent, categorical ratings to medications based on anticholinergic properties (1=low/minimal, 2=moderate, and 3=strong/definite).

Most of the total anticholinergic burden was attributable to antipsychotics, followed by "traditional" anticholinergics (eg, benztropine, diphenhydramine, hydroxyzine, and trihexyphenidyl), antidepressants, mood stabilizers, and benzodiazepines (see also "Anticholinergic Properties of Selected Psychotropics" table). Most patients (90%) were taking a second-generation antipsychotic, 18% were taking two antipsychotics, and 20% were taking benztropine or a similar medication.

RESULTS:

Greater anticholinergic burden was associated with significantly worse cognition scores after controlling for potential confounding factors, including dose and number of antipsychotics, psychotic symptom severity, illness duration, number of hospitalizations, and smoking. The global cognition of patients with high or very high anticholinergic burden was approximately 0.5 standard deviations below patients with no anticholinergic burden—meaning a moderate difference.

Limitations of this study included the cross-sectional design, which precludes causal inferences, and the exclusion of patients with significant medical conditions (leading to a likely underestimation of the impact of anticholinergic burden). Also, the ACB does not account for dose or previous medication exposures, or the effects of medication adherence.

CARLAT TAKE:
Anticholinergic medications may impair cognition in schizophrenia.

PRACTICE IMPLICATIONS:
Consider antipsychotics with a lower anticholinergic burden, particularly for patients who are elderly, have cognitive problems, or are taking other anticholinergic medications.

TABLE: Anticholinergic Properties of Selected Psychotropics

Class	ACB Score		
	Strong/Definite	Moderate	Low/Minimal
Second-generation antipsychotics	Clozapine Olanzapine Quetiapine		Aripiprazole Asenapine Iloperidone Lurasidone Paliperidone Risperidone Ziprasidone
First-generation antipsychotics	Chlorpromazine Fluphenazine Perphenazine Thioridazine Trifluoperazine	Loxapine Prochlorperazine Thiothixene	Haloperidol
Mood stabilizers		Carbamazepine Oxcarbazepine	Valproic acid
Antidepressants	Amitriptyline Clomipramine Doxepin Nortriptyline Paroxetine		Bupropion Citalopram Duloxetine Escitalopram Fluoxetine Fluvoxamine Mirtazapine Nefazodone Sertraline Trazodone Venlafaxine
Anticholinergics	Benztropine Diphenhydramine Hydroxyzine Trihexyphenidyl		

Source: www.acbcalc.com

Antidepressants Harm Some With Bipolar Depression

REVIEW OF: Ghaemi SN, Whitham EA, Vohringer PA, et al. Citalopram for Acute and Preventive Efficacy in Bipolar Depression (CAPE-BD): A randomized, double-blind, placebo-controlled trial. *J Clin Psychiatry*. 2021;82(1):19m13136.

STUDY TYPE: Randomized controlled trial

Antidepressants are controversial in bipolar depression, in part because we don't have enough well-designed studies to clarify their role. The most rigorous trials have come up negative, and many of the positive ones have suffered design flaws (eg, lack of placebo, small sample sizes, or enriched designs). On the other hand, few of these studies have uncovered significant rates of manic switching, as long as a mood stabilizer is on board. This new study adds weight to those findings as the first placebo-controlled trial to examine the long-term effects of an SSRI in bipolar disorder.

The National Institute of Mental Health–funded study randomized 119 patients with bipolar I or II depression to citalopram or placebo as an add-on to a "traditional" mood stabilizer ("traditional" means an antipsychotic was not allowed as the sole mood stabilizer but carbamazepine, lamotrigine, lithium, and valproate were). Citalopram was started at 10 mg/day and increased by 10 mg every week as needed toward a max of 60 mg/day (mean of 27 mg/day). Subjects were monitored using rating scales for depression and mania at six weeks (primary outcome) and one year (secondary outcome).

RESULTS:

Compared to placebo, citalopram brought no significant differences in response, remission, or change in depressive symptoms after acute (six week) and long-term (one year) follow-up. Likewise, there was no difference in manic symptoms or new episodes of hypomania or mania at either time point, and analysis of the month-by-month trend in symptoms also revealed no differences.

The authors then broke the data down by three bipolar subtypes: type I, type II, and rapid cycling. No differences emerged between types I and II, but those who entered the study with a recent history of rapid cycling (n=33) had significant worsening of manic symptoms (mean of 2-point increase over placebo on the MRS-SAD mania scale). The finding that an antidepressant did not help and may have harmed the rapid cycling group is supported by earlier studies.

The main weakness of this study was the dropout rate, which, although high (30% short term, 69% long term), was within the range seen in maintenance bipolar trials. These patients were handled conservatively with intention-to-treat analyses and were evenly distributed between the two groups. Most were patients who exited the trial because they required further therapeutic intervention for worsening symptoms.

CARLAT TAKE:

Whether you fall into the pro, con, or uncertain camp on antidepressants in bipolar disorder, this study suggests they are not very helpful for the average patient and—in line with earlier work—should be avoided for patients with rapid cycling.

PRACTICE IMPLICATIONS:

If you do prescribe an antidepressant in bipolar disorder, use it alongside a mood stabilizer and monitor carefully for rapid cycling with a mood chart. Rapid cycling is difficult to detect and includes patients who cycle in and out of depression without any manias, as long as there are at least four distinct episodes in a year.

Antipsychotic Dosing: How High?

REVIEW OF: Leucht S, Crippa A, Siafis S, Patel MX, Orsini N, Davis JM. Dose-response meta-analysis of antipsychotic drugs for acute schizophrenia. *Am J Psychiatry*. 2020;177(4):342–353. [Published correction appears in *Am J Psychiatry* 2020;177(3):272]

STUDY TYPE: Meta-analysis

How high should we go when dosing antipsychotics in schizophrenia? Surprisingly little is known about optimal doses. During drug development, dosing is estimated from animal studies, but more detailed studies in humans are rare. A 2020 meta-analysis of 68 studies examined dose-response relationships in randomized controlled trials of antipsychotic medications for schizophrenia and schizoaffective disorder. The outcome of interest was the dose producing a 95% reduction in symptoms (ED95).

RESULTS:

For many medications, the ED95 differed greatly from the FDA-recommended maximum. For example, aripiprazole's ED95 was 11.5 mg/day, in contrast to the 30 mg/day maximum licensed dose. For numerous medications (including clozapine, lurasidone, and olanzapine), the dose-response curves did not plateau, implying that dose escalation beyond the ED95 may still be efficacious. Other medications, such as brexpiprazole, cariprazine, and quetiapine, showed a clear plateau in dose response—implying no extra benefit of further escalation. Several medications showed a bell-shaped dose-response curve, including aripiprazole, haloperidol, and risperidone, implying a negative response with a higher dose.

TABLE: Dose-Response Relationships for Antipsychotic Drugs

	ED95 (mg/day)	FDA Max Licensed Dose (mg)	No Plateau (i.e., dose escalation beyond the ED95 may help)	Plateau (i.e., dose escalation beyond the ED95 provides no extra benefit)	Bell-Shaped (i.e., dose escalation beyond the ED95 worsens response)
Aripiprazole	12	30			X
Aripiprazole LAI (Lauroxil)	463 (q4wks)	882 (q4wks)		X	
Asenapine	15	20		X	
Brexpiprazole	3	4		X	
Cariprazine	8	6		X	
Clozapine	567	900	X		
Haloperidol	6	100			X
Iloperidone	20	24	X		
Lurasidone	147	160	X		

(table continues)

TABLE (CONTINUED): Dose-Response Relationships for Antipsychotic Drugs

	ED95 (mg/day)	FDA Max Licensed Dose (mg)	No Plateau (i.e., dose escalation beyond the ED95 may help)	Plateau (i.e., dose escalation beyond the ED95 provides no extra benefit)	Bell-Shaped (i.e., dose escalation beyond the ED95 worsens response)
Olanzapine, predominant negative symptoms	6	N/A			X
Olanzapine, predominant positive symptoms	15	20	X		
Olanzapine LAI	277 (q2wks)	300 (q2wks)	X		
Paliperidone	13	12	X		
Paliperidone LAI	120	234	X		
Quetiapine	482	IR: 750 ER: 800		X	
Risperidone	6	16			X
Risperidone LAI	37 (q2wks)	50			X
Sertindole	23	24	X		
Ziprasidone	186	200	X		

CARLAT TAKE:

For some commonly used agents, such as aripiprazole and quetiapine, we may be dosing patients more aggressively than needed. Serum drug levels can be obtained if a patient doesn't respond to the usual dose; this information can identify fast metabolizers for whom higher doses are needed.

PRACTICE IMPLICATIONS:

Dosing medications is always a matter of titrating for an individual patient. That said, this study may inform when we decide to augment or switch.

MANAGING ADVERSE EFFECTS

Antipsychotic Use Associated With Increased Risk of Mortality

REVIEW OF: Gerhard T, Stroup TS, Correll CU, et al. Mortality risk of antipsychotic augmentation for adult depression. *PLOS ONE.* 2020;15(9):e0239206.

STUDY TYPE: Population-based comparator cohort study

ATYPICAL ANTIPSYCHOTICS INCREASE mortality in elderly patients with dementia—the FDA has long required a black box warning to that effect. But are these medications also dangerous when prescribed to younger people with depression?

To try to answer this question, researchers analyzed mortality rates of depressed adults ages 25–64 enrolled in Medicaid between 2001 and 2010. Patients with major depression, but not other major Axis I disorders, who had failed to respond to at least three months of antidepressant monotherapy were included. The researchers compared two cohorts: patients who had their antidepressant augmented with an antipsychotic (n=22,410) versus those who had it augmented with a second antidepressant (n=17,172). The outcome of interest was all-cause mortality rates over the next year for patients who remained on their medications.

RESULTS:

In total, 105 deaths occurred during 7,601 person-years of follow-up in the antipsychotic cohort (138 per 100,000 person-years) versus 48 deaths during 5,727 person-years of follow-up in the antidepressant augmentation cohort (84 per 100,000 person-years). These numbers translate into an absolute risk of about 0.4% per year on antipsychotics, and a relative risk of 45% compared to antidepressant augmentation. To put this figure in perspective, the relative risk in elderly patients with dementia has been estimated to be 54%, which the FDA deemed concerning enough to trigger a black box warning. Among the four antipsychotics with sufficient sample sizes, olanzapine and risperidone were associated with the highest risks of mortality, while quetiapine and aripiprazole were associated with the lowest—findings that are consistent with geriatric research.

The main weakness of the study was the lack of randomization, leaving open the questions of which way the potential relationship might go and whether other factors are relevant. For example, clinicians might have chosen atypicals for more severely depressed patients. However, clinicians might have preferred antidepressant augmentation for patients with medical comorbidities, which would be expected to artificially inflate mortality rates in this cohort instead. We should also be cautious in generalizing results from Medicaid patients to the overall population.

CARLAT TAKE:

While this was only one study, and the increased mortality risk was small, the results should still give us pause before prescribing atypical antipsychotics in depression. It may be time to recalibrate their risk/benefit ratio.

PRACTICE IMPLICATIONS:

Especially for patients who have metabolic comorbidities, consider first augmenting antidepressants with other evidence-based treatments, such as transcranial magnetic stimulation, electroconvulsive therapy, lithium, thyroid hormone, or buspirone.

Beta-Blockers and Depression: The Controversy Revisited

REVIEW OF: Agustini B, Mohebbi M, Woods RL, et al. The association of antihypertensive use and depressive symptoms in a large older population with hypertension living in Australia and the United States: A cross-sectional study. *J Hum Hypertens*. 2020;34(11):787–794.

STUDY TYPE: Cross-sectional study

Antihypertensives are among the world's most widely prescribed drugs, but many of them impact pathways associated with depression. Beta-blockers have long been believed to cause depression, but most of these studies were carried out decades ago, and the findings have been inconsistent. Other classes, like angiotensin receptor blockers, are associated with lower rates of depression, albeit with weaker evidence.

In this multinational study, researchers examined mood outcomes in 14,195 hypertensive adults over 65 who did not have heart disease. Depressive symptoms were measured with the self-reported Centre for Epidemiological Studies-Depression (CESD-10) scale. Each class of antihypertensive drugs was tested against the other classes and against a group of unmedicated hypertensive patients to see whether any class was associated with an increased risk of clinically significant depressive symptoms.

RESULTS:

Patients who took beta-blockers were more likely to meet or exceed the cutoff of 8 on the CESD-10 scale, a sign of clinically significant depressive symptoms, than those who took other antihypertensive drugs. Numerically, 13.4% of patients who used beta-blockers showed clinical elevations in depression, whereas between 10.2% and 10.5% of patients who used other antihypertensives showed this elevation. Logistic regression analysis showed that this difference was indeed significant, even when controlling for numerous factors that included gender, age, and smoking history. Other classes of antihypertensives, including angiotensin receptor blockers, angiotensin-converting enzyme inhibitors, and calcium channel blockers, were not associated with depression.

The researchers also compared the beta-blockers based on their selectivity for the beta receptor and their lipophilic properties. Lipophilic medications are more likely to cross the blood-brain barrier, and the more lipophilic beta-blockers like propranolol and metoprolol were associated with a higher risk of depression than hydrophilic ones such as atenolol. Meanwhile, the less selective beta-blockers were less depressogenic, a finding that again favored atenolol.

CARLAT TAKE:
The fact that beta-blockers were associated with depression while other antihypertensives were not gives us pause, particularly with the widespread use of propranolol in psychiatry. The increase in depression was small but real in this large study of patients over 65.

PRACTICE IMPLICATIONS:
Psychiatric patients, especially those who are over 65 and have hypertension, will do best to avoid beta-blockers—or, if one must be used, stick with atenolol.

Comparison of GI Side Effects of Antidepressants

REVIEW OF: Oliva V, Lippi M, Paci R, et al. Gastrointestinal side effects associated with antidepressant treatments in patients with major depressive disorder: A systematic review and meta-analysis. *Prog Neuropsychopharmacol Biol Psychiatry*. 2021;109:110266.

STUDY TYPE: Meta-analysis

ANTIDEPRESSANTS OFTEN CAUSE gastrointestinal (GI) side effects, but it's not clear which are the worst offenders. A recent meta-analysis helps to clarify the picture.

The investigators searched the literature and located 304 randomized, placebo-controlled trials with information on GI side effects related to 15 antidepressants, including SSRIs, SNRIs, bupropion, and mirtazapine.

RESULTS:

Nausea and vomiting were the most common side effect, with the five worst offenders being duloxetine (odds ratio [OR] 4.33), vortioxetine (OR 4.28), levomilnacipran (OR 3.81), venlafaxine (OR 3.52), and desvenlafaxine (OR 3.51). Only mirtazapine was not associated with nausea and vomiting, which is consistent with its mechanism of action. The risk of nausea and vomiting was dose dependent for citalopram and escitalopram and became more pronounced at dosages above 40 mg/day for citalopram and 10 mg/day for escitalopram.

Constipation was associated with 10 antidepressants, with levomilnacipran (OR 3.41), desvenlafaxine (OR 3.41), and duloxetine (OR 2.58) the top three. Vortioxetine had a dose-dependent risk of constipation at dosages above the maximum recommended dose of 20 mg/day. Five antidepressants were associated with diarrhea: sertraline (OR 2.33), fluvoxamine (OR 2.29), escitalopram (OR 1.91), citalopram (OR 1.64), and duloxetine (OR 1.60).

Other GI side effects were also examined (see "Gastrointestinal Side Effects Examined" table).

TABLE: Gastrointestinal Side Effects Examined

Side Effect	Antidepressants Most Likely to Cause (ordered from more to less likely)
Nausea/vomiting	Duloxetine, vortioxetine, levomilnacipran, venlafaxine, desvenlafaxine
Constipation	Levomilnacipran, desvenlafaxine, duloxetine
Diarrhea	Sertraline, fluvoxamine, escitalopram, citalopram, duloxetine
Abdominal pain	Escitalopram and citalopram
Anorexia	Fluvoxamine, desvenlafaxine, venlafaxine, paroxetine, duloxetine
Increased appetite	Mirtazapine

CARLAT TAKE:

While most antidepressants can cause GI side effects, it appears that SNRIs and vortioxetine are the most likely to cause both nausea and constipation. True to its reputation, sertraline caused the most diarrhea. Paroxetine was associated with anorexia, suggesting this medication may have opposite effects in different patients, as other studies have associated it with weight gain. Surprisingly, the two antidepressants associated with weight loss—bupropion and fluoxetine—did not decrease patients' appetite in this meta-analysis.

PRACTICE IMPLICATIONS:

The more we can quantify the most likely side effect profile for differing medications, the more we can tailor our decision-making and risk/benefit discussions with patients. For example, SNRIs may not be the best first-line options for patients who are already prone to nausea or constipation.

Do Structural Brain Abnormalities Predict Cognitive Impairment With Electroconvulsive Therapy?

REVIEW OF: Wagenmakers MJ, Vansteelandt K, van Exel E, et al. Transient cognitive impairment and white matter hyperintensities in severely depressed older patients treated with electroconvulsive therapy. *Am J Geriatr Psychiatry*. 2021;29(11):1117–1128.

STUDY TYPE: Prospective observational study

We know that a subset of patients with late-life depression who are treated with electroconvulsive therapy (ECT) develop transient cognitive impairment (TCI). Is there any way to predict which patients will experience the most memory loss? Some studies have linked white matter hyperintensities (WMH), which represent brain damage generally associated with small-vessel disease, with an increased risk for TCI in ECT patients (Oudega ML et al, *Am J Geriatr Psychiatry* 2014;22(2):157–166). This study investigated associations between WMH, medial temporal lobe atrophy (MTA), or global cortical atrophy (GCA), and TCI following ECT.

Eighty elderly patients with severe unipolar depression were followed before and after a course of ECT. All patients started with right unilateral ECT, although approximately one-third required a switch to bilateral ECT due to clinical worsening. Patients had a median age of 73 years, and 67.5% were female. All received an MRI, and cognitive functioning was assessed before and after ECT with the Mini-Mental State Exam (MMSE). Patients with comorbid psychiatric and neurological illness (including dementia) were excluded.

RESULTS:

Although MMSE scores dropped for all participants by an average of two points during ECT, MMSE scores improved above baseline post-ECT by two to three points, and remained stable six months later, independent of structural brain abnormalities. Patients with severe WMH had lower scores at all stages compared to patients without severe WMH, but the trajectory was similar for both groups. Regardless of the brain finding (WMH, MTA, or GCA), there was no significant association with degree of cognitive impairment.

CARLAT TAKE:
We often worry about the effects of ECT on cognition, especially in patients with known structural brain abnormalities. This study is encouraging, as cognition returned to baseline levels post-ECT independent of the severity of WMH, MTA, or GCA.

PRACTICE IMPLICATIONS:
ECT is the most effective treatment for late-life depression, and we can continue to recommend ECT in patients with these specific structural brain impairments.

Lithium Exposure In Utero: How Bad Is It Really?

REVIEW OF: Fornaro M, Maritan E, Ferranti R, et al. Lithium exposure during pregnancy and the postpartum period: A systematic review and meta-analysis of safety and efficacy outcomes. *Am J Psychiatry*. 2020;177(1):76–92.

STUDY TYPE: Systematic review and meta-analysis

Most of us are wary of prescribing lithium to pregnant women, but is prenatal lithium exposure as risky as we think? A meta-analysis of 13 case-control, cohort, and interventional studies involving 1,349,563 pregnancies compared congenital anomalies among lithium-exposed and unexposed mothers with and without bipolar disorder.

RESULTS:

Lithium use at any time in pregnancy, compared with unexposed women (either women with bipolar disorder or general population controls), was associated with a significantly elevated risk of congenital and cardiac anomalies (odds ratio [OR] 1.75; 95% CI [1.23, 2.48]; p<0.01 and OR 1.86; 95% CI [1.16, 2.96]; p<0.01, respectively). The risks were higher if lithium was used in the first trimester and for higher doses and serum levels. The rate of cardiac malformations tripled with dosages above 900 mg/day when compared with dosages under 600 mg/day or maternal lithium levels below 0.64 mEq/L. At these lower doses, the risk of cardiac malformations was comparable to that of unexposed newborns. The absolute risks of anomalies were relatively low: 4.2% for any malformation, and 1.2% for cardiac malformations.

First-trimester lithium exposure was also linked with a higher risk of spontaneous abortion (OR 3.77; 95% CI [1.15, 12.39]; p=0.03)—but this risk was about the same in pregnant women with mood disorders not on lithium. This suggests that the underlying mood disorder contributes to the risk of spontaneous abortion. Infants exposed to lower lithium doses were noted to be more reactive.

Surprisingly, compared to no lithium use, lithium was not more effective at preventing a postpartum mood relapse.

The authors pointed out several limitations in their data, including a lack of information on other prescribed medications besides lithium.

CARLAT TAKE:

Lithium use during pregnancy, especially in the first trimester, elevates the risks of congenital and cardiac anomalies, but lithium also helps prevent postpartum mood relapses. While this study has methodological limitations typically inherent in research on prenatal psychotropic medication exposures, it provides helpful guidelines for the use of lithium in pregnant women.

PRACTICE IMPLICATIONS:

Whenever feasible, avoid or minimize in utero lithium exposure, especially in the first trimester. Nevertheless, the absolute risk of congenital anomalies remains low—and you can reduce this risk further by keeping the lithium dose below 600 mg/day and the maternal lithium levels below 0.64 mEq/L. However, some patients, especially those with severe illness, may require higher lithium concentrations to remain stable.

MANAGING ADVERSE EFFECTS

New Combination Treatment Mitigates Antipsychotic-Induced Weight Gain

REVIEW OF: Correll CU, Newcomer JW, Silverman B, et al. Effects of olanzapine combined with samidorphan on weight gain in schizophrenia: A 24-week Phase 3 study. *Am J Psychiatry.* 2020;177(12):1168–1178.

STUDY TYPE: Randomized controlled trial

Before olanzapine/samidorphan (Lybalvi) was approved by the FDA for schizophrenia and bipolar disorder in 2021, we had no on-label medications to mitigate antipsychotic-associated weight gain.

In this 24-week, double-blind trial, 352 adults with schizophrenia were randomized to receive either olanzapine alone (n=176) or a combination tablet of olanzapine and samidorphan, an opioid antagonist (n=176). Olanzapine doses were 10 or 20 mg daily; samidorphan was 10 mg daily. Alkermes, the manufacturer of the combination drug, sponsored the study. Exclusion criteria were strict and included treatment-resistant schizophrenia, substance use disorders, any clinically significant medical illness (eg, diabetes, hypertension), obesity (BMI greater than 30), and recent use of opioids or opioid antagonists.

RESULTS:

At the 24-week endpoint of the study, patients on olanzapine/samidorphan gained 4.2% of their body weight, significantly less than the 6.6% gained by those taking olanzapine alone. Other key outcomes favoring olanzapine/samidorphan included the proportion of subjects who gained more than 10% of their baseline body weight (olanzapine/samidorphan 18% vs olanzapine 30%) and the mean change in baseline waist circumference (olanzapine/samidorphan 2.4 cm vs olanzapine 4.5 cm). Metabolic changes were minimal for both groups. Dropout rates were primarily associated with adverse events, impacting 12% of the combined-treatment group and 9.8% of the olanzapine group.

The most common adverse events were weight gain and increased appetite (more in the olanzapine-only group), and somnolence and dry mouth (more in the combined-treatment group). The addition of samidorphan did not affect antipsychotic efficacy. About one-third of patients dropped out due to side effects, loss to follow-up, or unspecified reasons.

CARLAT TAKE:

Especially for inpatients, it is unusual to find patients with schizophrenia who do not have a substance use problem, a significant medical problem, or recent use of opioids or opioid antagonists, so we don't know if these findings apply to our typical patients. Lybalvi is brand-name only and may be too expensive for many patients, and samidorphan is not available as a stand-alone prescription to combine with generic olanzapine. Given how problematic antipsychotic-induced weight gain can be for our patients, Lybalvi may become a useful tool, but you can also consider off-label metformin if Lybalvi is not affordable or is contraindicated.

PRACTICE IMPLICATIONS:

Adding samidorphan to olanzapine appeared to decrease weight gain for adults with schizophrenia, but the effect was only moderate. To put this in perspective, a patient starting the trial at 150 pounds would have gained an average of 9.9 pounds on olanzapine versus 6.3 pounds on the combination.

Omega-3s and Metabolic Risks in Schizophrenia

REVIEW OF: Pawełczyk T, Grancow-Grabka M, Żurner N, Pawełczyk A. Omega-3 fatty acids reduce cardiometabolic risk in first-episode schizophrenia patients treated with antipsychotics: Findings from the OFFER randomized controlled study. *Schizophr Res*. 2021;230:61–68.

STUDY TYPE: Randomized controlled trial

Patients with schizophrenia are at greater risk for metabolic syndrome, whether from lifestyle, antipsychotic side effects, or the illness itself. Omega-3 fatty acids have metabolic benefits in the general population, and levels of these "healthy fats" tend to be low in people with schizophrenia. Earlier research found that omega-3 supplementation improved negative symptoms in schizophrenia, and this study examined their metabolic effects in schizophrenia.

This was a small, randomized, double-blind, placebo-controlled trial of 71 adults with stable schizophrenia on antipsychotic medication. They were treated with either omega-3 fatty acids or a fish-flavored placebo for six months. Both the placebo and the active intervention contained 0.2% alpha-tocopherol (vitamin E) to prevent oxidation of fatty acids. The omega-3 intervention consisted of a 3:1 ratio of eicosapentaenoic (EPA) and docosahexaenoic (DHA) acids with a total daily dosage of 2.2 mg. Body composition and metabolic parameters associated with metabolic syndrome were assessed at baseline, eight weeks, and 26 weeks after study initiation. Both groups began the trial with similar metabolic parameters.

RESULTS:

After eight weeks, the placebo group had a nonsignificant increase in metabolic syndrome (p=0.083), and this increase was even greater, and significant, at 26 weeks (p=0.007). By contrast, the rate of metabolic syndrome decreased in the treatment group (p=0.0408). Notably, the omega-3 group had significant reductions in fasting blood glucose (p=0.045), total cholesterol (p=0.037), and blood glucose levels (p=0.034). Improvements of other metabolic parameters were not significant. Patients on olanzapine experienced the greatest metabolic benefits with omega-3s.

The investigators also found an association between triglyceride levels and the psychopathology subscale of the Positive and Negative Syndrome Scale, suggesting that lower triglycerides are associated with improved symptoms of psychopathology (p=0.0008).

Omega-3s were well tolerated in this study. They have a mild anticoagulant effect, but patients on anticoagulants can still take omega-3s with approval from the physician prescribing them. Omega-3 supplementation may deplete vitamin E, and this study gave a vitamin E supplement to avoid that.

CARLAT TAKE:

This study was small and preliminary, but omega-3s have established benefits for metabolic health in various conditions and are worth considering in schizophrenia. The 3:1 EPA:DHA ratio used in this study can be difficult to find but is worth the search, as this is also the ratio that has worked in studies of depression. We found three products with a similar ratio that were tested by independent labs: Viva Naturals (on Amazon), Member's Mark (at Sam's Club), and Kirkland Signature (at Costco) at a cost of 15–25 cents/day. Vascepa, which is FDA approved for elevated triglycerides, also has a high ratio of EPA.

PRACTICE IMPLICATIONS:

On an intuitive level, diet and exercise seem like reasonable first steps for metabolic side effects of antipsychotics. On a practical level, they are difficult for patients to implement and become more difficult as weight gain increases. Omega-3 fatty acids will appeal to patients who prefer a natural approach, and the FDA-approved Vascepa alleviates concerns around product reliability. Omega-3s' additional benefits for negative symptoms of schizophrenia are the icing on the fish cake.

Polypharmacy in Schizophrenia

REVIEW OF: Tiihonen J, Taipale H, Mehtälä J, Vattulainen P, Correll CU, Tanskanen A. Association of antipsychotic polypharmacy vs monotherapy with psychiatric rehospitalization among adults with schizophrenia. *JAMA Psychiatry*. 2019;76(5):499–507.

Stroup TS, Gerhard T, Crystal S, et al. Comparative effectiveness of adjunctive psychotropic medications in patients with schizophrenia. *JAMA Psychiatry*. 2019;76(5):508–515.

STUDY TYPES: Two retrospective, non-randomized, controlled trials

Antipsychotic polypharmacy is discouraged in guidelines but common in practice. Up to 30% of patients with schizophrenia are prescribed multiple antipsychotics, and combinations of antipsychotics with other drug classes are even more common. Research on these practices is sparse. Recently, two large retrospective, non-randomized, controlled trials attempted to clarify whether polypharmacy brings greater benefits in schizophrenia or just greater risks.

The first study collected data from a population-wide registry in Finland of 62,250 patients with schizophrenia who were hospitalized and followed between 1996 and 2015 (median age 46; male to female ratio equal).

Hazard ratios (HRs) were calculated by comparing patients on one, multiple, or no antipsychotics. Within-individual analysis was used to eliminate selection bias (ie, each patient was their own control). Of the total cohort, 67% used antipsychotic polypharmacy at some point. To exclude switches between antipsychotics, data from the first 90 days of multiple antipsychotic use were censored. The primary outcome was psychiatric rehospitalization, and secondary outcomes were mortality and medical hospitalization.

The second study evaluated the effects of adding different drug classes to standard treatment in schizophrenia. Using a Medicaid registry, 81,921 patients with schizophrenia on antipsychotic therapy were followed for one year after starting an additional psychotropic (mean age 41; 54% male). Patients who were already on multiple psychiatric medications or who filled their antipsychotic inconsistently were excluded from the sample (n=241 and 579 respectively).

HRs were calculated comparing patients based on whether they were prescribed antidepressants, benzodiazepines, or mood stabilizers vs additional antipsychotics. Patients in each of the treatment groups were demographically similar. Those who did not start a new psychotropic were not included in the comparisons, as it was thought they represented a group with fewer comorbidities and better prognoses. Dropouts were handled by analyzing data on an intent-to-treat basis. The primary outcome was psychiatric hospitalization, and secondary outcomes included mortality and medical hospitalization.

RESULTS:

In the first study, the risk of psychiatric rehospitalization was 13% lower with polypharmacy than monotherapy (HR 0.87; 95% CI [0.85, 0.88]). That risk was lowest with the combination of clozapine and aripiprazole: 58% lower than no antipsychotic use (HR 0.42; 95% CI [0.39, 0.46]) and 14% lower than clozapine alone (HR 0.86; 95% CI [0.79, 0.94]). Among the top 10 treatments with the lowest risk of rehospitalization, only one was monotherapy: clozapine. Remarkably, polypharmacy was also associated with a lower risk of hospitalization due to medical illness and mortality.

In the second study, the risk of psychiatric hospitalization was 16% lower for patients who started an antidepressant (HR 0.84; 95% CI [0.80, 0.88]). Patients started on benzodiazepines had a higher risk of psychiatric hospitalization (HR 1.08; 95% CI [1.02, 1.15]), while those started on mood stabilizers had an equal risk (HR 0.98; 95% CI [0.94, 1.03]). Antidepressants were associated with a lower risk of medical hospitalization (HR 0.87; 95% CI [0.79, 0.96]), whereas no difference was found for benzodiazepines or mood stabilizers. Mood stabilizers were the only group associated with a statistically higher risk of mortality (HR 1.31; 95% CI [1.04, 1.66]), and this risk was highest with gabapentin.

Both studies had similar weaknesses. With the lack of randomization, various confounding variables could have been overlooked. Factors not examined include reasons for changing medications, frequency of patient-provider contact, use of psychosocial interventions, and extent of medication adherence. Functioning and symptom severity were also not examined. On the other hand, patients prescribed multiple psychotropics are likely to have lower functioning and greater disease severity, so it is impressive that these patients had favorable outcomes.

CARLAT TAKE:
When combining antipsychotics, the best outcome was with clozapine and aripiprazole. This suggests that prescribing antipsychotics with different receptor profiles may be a useful tactic. In terms of combining antipsychotics with other psychotropics, the results are less definitive. Antidepressants appear to have the greatest benefit and least risk; mood stabilizers and benzodiazepines should be used with more caution.

PRACTICE IMPLICATIONS:
Polypharmacy is a viable strategy for some patients with schizophrenia who do not respond to antipsychotic monotherapy. On the other hand, it brings additional risks and should only be used after careful attempts to titrate off prove unworkable.

A Single Prescriber Reduces Risk of Overdose in Patients on Opioids and Benzodiazepines

REVIEW OF: Chua KP, Brummett CM, Ng S, Bohnert ASB. Association between receipt of overlapping opioid and benzodiazepine prescriptions from multiple prescribers and overdose risk. *JAMA Netw Open*. 2021;4(8):e2120353.

STUDY TYPE: Retrospective cohort analysis

When a patient on an opioid requires a benzodiazepine, should the two medications be handled by the same prescriber or by separate prescribers? Among patients on opioids, one in five are also prescribed a benzodiazepine, but the combination raises the risk of opioid overdose fatalities fourfold. This study was the first to look at safety outcomes for single versus multiple prescribers.

Using a database of medical and pharmacy claims, researchers performed a retrospective cohort analysis, identifying patients who had one or more days of benzodiazepine-opioid overlap between January 1, 2017, and December 31, 2018. Ultimately, the cohort included 529,053 patients ages 12 years and older, with an average age of 61. Researchers determined whether the opioids and benzodiazepines were prescribed by a single clinician or by two or more clinicians. The primary outcome measure was the occurrence of an overdose.

RESULTS:

The relative overdose risk, adjusted for prescribing patterns, demographics, and comorbidities, was 1.2 times greater when benzodiazepine-opioid overlap involved multiple prescribers vs a single prescriber (unadjusted overdose risk was 1.8 times greater). This translates to a 20% increased risk of overdose.

CARLAT TAKE:
Benzodiazepine and opioid combinations are risky, but the risk goes down when one clinician monitors both scripts. This study can't tell us why, but it's likely easier to detect problematic use with that arrangement via urine drug screen results and pill counts.

PRACTICE IMPLICATIONS:
For your patients taking both a benzodiazepine and an opioid, consolidate prescribers. For most psychiatrists, this probably means deferring benzo prescriptions to the opioid prescriber.

Vitamin B$_6$ Lowers Prolactin on Antipsychotics

REVIEW OF: Zhuo C, Xu Y, Wang H, et al. Safety and efficacy of high-dose vitamin B6 as an adjunctive treatment for antipsychotic-induced hyperprolactinemia in male patients with treatment-resistant schizophrenia. *Front Psychiatry*. 2021;12:681418.

STUDY TYPE: Randomized controlled trial

Hyperprolactinemia, a common side effect of antipsychotics, can cause multiple issues, including sexual dysfunction and gynecomastia. It is a particular problem in treatment-resistant schizophrenia: Patients often need higher antipsychotic doses, which are more likely to elevate prolactin. Dopamine agonists like bromocriptine can reverse the effect, as can low doses of the dopamine partial agonist aripiprazole (that's right, this antipsychotic actually treats hyperprolactinemia)—but beyond that, there is limited evidence for other treatment options. Vitamin B$_6$ showed potential in earlier research, and this study tested that treatment in a large, controlled trial.

This was a randomized, double-blind trial in China that tested high-dose vitamin B$_6$ against an active control (low-dose aripiprazole) in 200 adult males ages 20–40 with treatment-resistant schizophrenia and hyperprolactinemia. Patients received either aripiprazole 5 mg twice daily or vitamin B$_6$ 300 mg twice daily, in addition to their current antipsychotic, for 16 weeks. Patients randomized to vitamin B$_6$ were much younger, had higher education, and had significantly higher prolactin levels at baseline (95.5 vs 89.1 μg/L) than the aripiprazole group. Hyperprolactinemia was defined as a prolactin level greater than 25 μg/L, which is the usual cutoff for this hormone. Prolactin levels, psychotic symptoms, and cognition were assessed at baseline and every four weeks after study initiation. In total, 97% of subjects completed the trial.

RESULTS:

After 16 weeks, the vitamin B$_6$ group showed a much greater reduction in prolactin levels compared to the aripiprazole group (68.1% vs 37.4%). Both groups showed steep reductions in prolactin levels from baseline to week four, but the efficacy of aripiprazole plateaued after week eight, whereas vitamin B$_6$ further reduced prolactin levels through week 16. Furthermore, after 16 weeks, the vitamin B$_6$ group showed a greater reduction in psychotic symptoms (17.8% vs 12.0%) and improvement in cognition (10% vs -5.4%) compared with the aripiprazole group. Vitamin B$_6$ was well tolerated in this study, with fewer side effects than in the aripiprazole group. Vitamin B$_6$ also had favorable metabolic effects, as it did not increase blood glucose or lipids.

Limitations of this study include the fact that all subjects were male and had treatment-resistant schizophrenia. Therefore, the generalizability of findings to other patients and phases of illness is limited.

CARLAT TAKE:

Vitamin B$_6$ may be a viable treatment option for antipsychotic-induced hyperprolactinemia, at least in treatment-resistant schizophrenia. This study was included in a 2022 network meta-analysis that further confirmed vitamin B$_6$'s ability to lower prolactin levels (Lu Z et al, *Transl Psychiatry* 2022;12(1):267).

PRACTICE IMPLICATIONS:

Vitamin B$_6$ lowers prolactin on antipsychotics and may improve positive and negative symptoms of schizophrenia as well.

MOOD DISORDERS

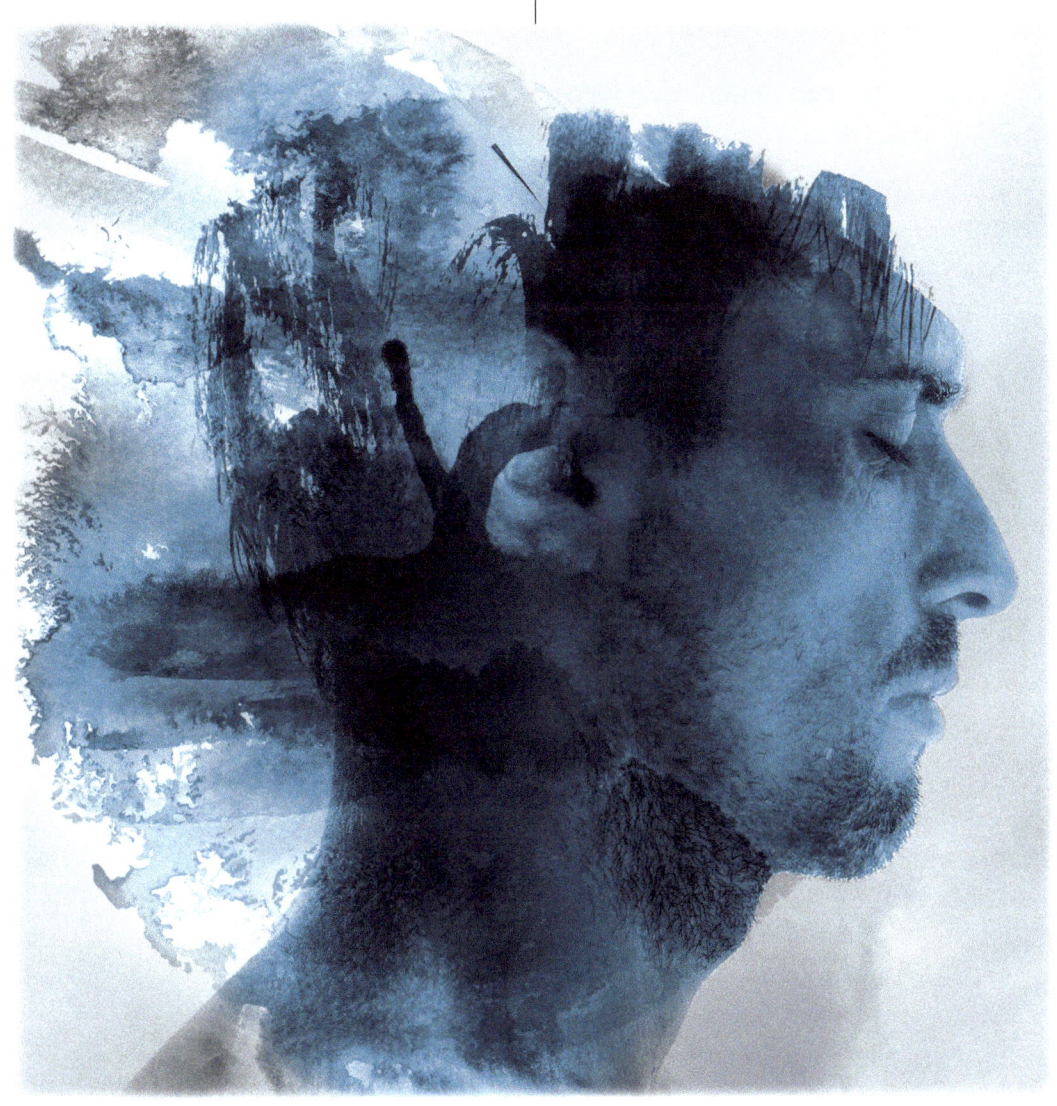

An Answer for Psychotic Depression

REVIEW OF: Flint AJ, Meyers BS, Rothschild AJ, et al. Effect of continuing olanzapine vs placebo on relapse among patients with psychotic depression in remission: The STOP-PD II randomized clinical trial. *JAMA*. 2019;322(7):622–631.

STUDY TYPE: Randomized controlled trial

Psychotic features in depression indicate a more severe form of the disease, with a higher risk of hospitalization and double the rate of disability compared with non-psychotic depression. A combination of an antipsychotic and an antidepressant is the mainstay of treatment, but how long to continue the antipsychotic is an unanswered question.

This study enrolled patients ages 18–85 years with severe major depression and at least one delusion; hallucinations were an optional criterion. Exclusion criteria included dementia and unstable medical illness. Average age was 55 years.

Researchers first treated 269 patients with open-label olanzapine and sertraline. Next, 162 patients who achieved remission or near-remission entered an open-label eight-week stabilization phase. Of the 147 who remained well after the eight-week stabilization, 126 were randomized to continue on olanzapine or have the antipsychotic replaced with a placebo for 36 weeks. This portion of the study was double-blinded, and the antipsychotic taper took place over four weeks. All patients remained on sertraline throughout the trial. The primary outcome was risk of relapse, which included relapses into depression or psychosis, as well as psychiatric hospitalization or suicidality.

RESULTS:

Relapses occurred in 55% of placebo patients, compared to 20% of olanzapine patients. The number needed to treat to keep patients well with continued antipsychotic therapy was 2.8. The majority of these relapses (79%) occurred within the first 20 weeks of the 36-week randomization phase.

Weight gain was the main side effect of continuing olanzapine. The placebo group lost weight, while the olanzapine group continued to gain, with a difference of 9 pounds between them at the end of the study. Falls were also greater in the olanzapine-continuation group (31% vs 18%).

CARLAT TAKE:

Given the exclusion criteria, this study's patients may not have been as ill as some whom we see in clinical practice. However, these results support continuing both antipsychotic and antidepressant therapies for patients recovering from psychotic depression.

PRACTICE IMPLICATIONS:

When treating psychotic depression with an antipsychotic and antidepressant, continue both for at least two months as long as they are reasonably tolerable. After six months of remission (28 weeks), consider a slow taper of the antipsychotic, taking into account the severity of the episode, side effects, and the patient's preferences.

Antidepressants for Suicidal Ideation in Depressed Patients?

REVIEW OF: Dunlop BW, Polychroniou PE, Rakofsky JJ, Nemeroff CB, Craighead WE, Mayberg HS. Suicidal ideation and other persisting symptoms after CBT or antidepressant medication treatment for major depressive disorder. *Psychol Med*. 2019;49(11):1869–1878.

STUDY TYPE: Post-hoc analysis of a randomized controlled trial

Antidepressants and cognitive behavioral therapy (CBT) appear roughly equivalent for treating depression (Weitz ES et al, *JAMA Psychiatry* 2015;72(11):1102–1109), but might they differ in their efficacy for individual symptoms of depression, such as insomnia, decreased appetite, or suicidal ideation (SI)?

To explore this question, researchers randomized 315 depressed adults to either 12 weeks of CBT or medication treatment (escitalopram or duloxetine). They used the Montgomery-Åsberg Depression Rating Scale (MADRS) to identify residual symptoms in the 250 subjects who completed the study (110 with severe depression and 140 with moderate depression). Subjects were categorized as responders if their MADRS score dropped by more than half during treatment. Residual symptoms from the CBT and medication groups were compared for each MADRS item, and residual symptoms of responders were compared to nonresponders.

RESULTS:

About two-thirds of the subjects were treatment responders (59% in the CBT group and 69% in the medication group), and residual symptoms, as measured by MADRS items, were comparable between CBT and medication groups. However, among the nonresponders, CBT subjects' mean score on SI rose by 15%, while it dropped by 70% in the medication group—ie, even when patients failed to respond to antidepressants, their suicidal thoughts diminished.

CARLAT TAKE:
Although both CBT and medications were effective for depression in this study, among treatment nonresponders, antidepressants significantly reduced SI even among patients who remained depressed. CBT had the opposite effect, with SI increasing among nonresponders.

PRACTICE IMPLICATIONS:
Medications appeared more effective than therapy in this study, even for depressed patients who failed to respond adequately, as the antidepressants reduced suicidal thoughts in medication nonresponders. These findings are worth keeping in mind when seeing patients with depression and suicidality.

Aripiprazole in Depression: The Right Dose

REVIEW OF: Furukawa Y, Hamza T, Cipriani A, Furukawa TA, Salanti G, Ostinelli EG. Optimal dose of aripiprazole for augmentation therapy of antidepressant-refractory depression: Preliminary findings based on a systematic review and dose-effect meta-analysis. *Br J Psychiatry*. 2022;221(2):440–447.

STUDY TYPE: Meta-analysis

Aripiprazole is FDA approved for antidepressant augmentation, and although it is the best studied atypical antipsychotic for this condition, dosing has not been nailed down. Guidelines recommend 2–15 mg/day, but higher doses bring additional risks like akathisia, sedation, and metabolic problems. This meta-analysis aimed to find the optimal dose range.

The authors found 10 double-blind, placebo-controlled, randomized studies in which aripiprazole was added to an SSRI or SNRI antidepressant in patients with treatment-resistant depression. The definition of treatment resistance varied among the studies, which required an inadequate response to one to three antidepressant trials lasting at least six to 12 weeks. Patients with other psychiatric and substance use disorders were excluded, as were any who had received electroconvulsive therapy in the last 10 years or had been on adjunctive antipsychotics in the last three weeks before starting aripiprazole.

These criteria yielded 2,625 patients, 55% female. Over half the studies took place in North America and about a third took place in Japan. Some of the studies compared augmentation with aripiprazole using a fixed-dose schedule, and some allowed flexible dosing. Trials lasted six to eight weeks. Doses ranged from 2 to 20 mg/day. Reduction in the Montgomery-Åsberg Depression Rating Scale (MADRS) was the main outcome measure. Tolerability (dropouts due to adverse effects) and acceptability (dropouts for any reason) were also tracked.

RESULTS:

The main finding was that efficacy was associated with doses between 2 and 5 mg, with no additional benefits at higher doses. Aripiprazole 4 mg resulted in a 36% improvement compared with 23% placebo response. Odds ratio of response gradually increased as doses increased from 2 mg (1.46) to 4 mg (1.87) and leveled off at 5 mg (1.91). Doses beyond 5 mg were well tolerated but didn't add clinical benefit.

CARLAT TAKE:

One limitation of this analysis was that it involved multiple studies with varied doses that were not designed to test the hypothesis at hand. It remains possible that some patients will do better at higher doses of adjunctive aripiprazole, but it is difficult to say who they are.

PRACTICE IMPLICATIONS:

When using aripiprazole for antidepressant augmentation, 2–5 mg is the ideal range.

Brexpiprazole Does Not Treat Mania

REVIEW OF: Vieta E, Sachs G, Chang D, et al. Two randomized, double-blind, placebo-controlled trials and one open-label, long-term trial of brexpiprazole for the acute treatment of bipolar mania. *J Psychopharmacol.* 2021;35(8):971–982.

STUDY TYPE: Two randomized controlled trials

Brexpiprazole is FDA approved in schizophrenia and as an adjunct for major depression, and is one of the better-tolerated antipsychotics. Like aripiprazole, it is a partial D2 and 5-HT1A agonist. Unlike most antipsychotics, brexpiprazole has never been studied in acute mania, so these two industry-sponsored trials gave us the first glimpse of its antimanic potential.

The two trials were large, randomized, placebo-controlled trials comparing brexpiprazole with placebo over three weeks in acute bipolar I mania. The participants were drawn from multiple US and European sites and had severe mania, with a Young Mania Rating Scale (YMRS) score over 24 at entry. Brexpiprazole was started at 2 mg/day and titrated up to 4 mg/day as tolerated. No other medication was allowed, except as-needed lorazepam. The trials enrolled 654 patients, and over 75% of them completed the acute phase.

RESULTS:

After three weeks, YMRS scores were about the same for drug and placebo, although the brexpiprazole group did score a little better on the secondary Clinical Global Impressions-Bipolar Disorder (CGI-BP) measure.

Both trials included an open-label, long-term phase where symptoms were treated with brexpiprazole for another six months if the investigators thought patients would benefit from continued treatment. This phase showed gradual decreases in YMRS and CGI-BP scores, but the changes were not dramatic and there was no control arm to compare them to.

Brexpiprazole was well tolerated, with akathisia the most commonly reported adverse effect. During the open-label extension, six patients became manic, five became depressed, and four developed suicidal ideation; again, these events lacked a placebo arm for comparison.

The multicenter design may have obscured a drug-placebo difference. There are more investigators per patient in multicenter trials, increasing the attention each patient receives and potentially amplifying any placebo effect. However, other antipsychotics have yielded positive results for mania in multicenter trials.

The industry-funded authors conducted a secondary analysis in an attempt to salvage some signal of response in these patients. Based on earlier evidence that poor insight predicts a better response to antipsychotics in mania (Welten CC et al, *J Clin Psychopharmacol.* 2016;36(1):71–76), they reanalyzed the data and found that poorer insight was associated with a statistically significant improvement on brexpiprazole relative to placebo (odds ratio 2.2; 95% CI [1.1, 4.4]).

CARLAT TAKE:

The atypical antipsychotics are a varied class, and we can't conclude all of them work in acute mania.

PRACTICE IMPLICATIONS:

When using antipsychotics in mania, stick with our FDA-approved antimanic agents: aripiprazole, cariprazine, olanzapine, risperidone, quetiapine, and ziprasidone. The others in this class are either untested (lurasidone and lumateperone) or have negative results in this condition (brexpiprazole and paliperidone).

Can Antidepressants Prolong Survival in Cancer Patients?

REVIEW OF: Shoval G, Balicer RD, Feldman B, et al. Adherence to antidepressant medications is associated with reduced premature mortality in patients with cancer: A nationwide cohort study. *Depress Anxiety.* 2019;36(10):921–929.

STUDY TYPE: Retrospective cohort study

Many cancer patients experience depression, especially those with poor prognoses. Compared with euthymic patients, depressed cancer patients are less adherent to their cytotoxic medications, and this poor adherence can worsen their long-term survival. Yet, surprisingly, some studies have reported a higher mortality rate among cancer patients taking antidepressants. Might confounding factors account for this finding (eg, patients with worse prognoses are more likely to be depressed and therefore to be placed on antidepressants)?

This large (n=42,075) retrospective cohort study controlled for several confounding factors to get a better understanding of the relationship between antidepressant use and mortality. Using an Israeli national health services database, the authors extracted data on patients who were diagnosed with cancer and who purchased an antidepressant prescription within the four-year study period (2008–2012). Patients were further divided into subgroups based on antidepressant adherence, ranging from non-adherent to highly adherent. Adherence was defined as the number of months with actual filled prescriptions divided by the number of months when an antidepressant was prescribed.

RESULTS:

An initial analysis indicated an increase in mortality with antidepressant adherence, but also revealed that older and sicker patients tended to be the most adherent, leading to an overrepresentation of mortality in the adherent group.

A subsequent analysis, adjusting for such factors, showed the opposite: Antidepressant-adherent patients lived significantly longer than minimally adherent (<20% adherence) or non-adherent patients. The mortality rate among patients with the highest antidepressant adherence (>80% adherence) was 20% lower over the four-year study period, compared to the minimally adherent or non-adherent groups. Subgroup analyses showed this adherence benefit remained regardless of cancer type, including lung, prostate, breast, and colon.

CARLAT TAKE:
This large retrospective study found that antidepressant adherence was associated with improved survival in people with cancer. Whether this was due to greater adherence to cancer treatment or some other reason remains unclear. Further studies with psychotherapy controls may provide additional insights.

PRACTICE IMPLICATIONS:
We should assess and treat depression in cancer patients and encourage medication adherence.

Can We Treat Depression by Targeting Inflammation?

REVIEW OF: Zazula R, Husain MI, Mohebbi M, et al. Minocycline as adjunctive treatment for major depressive disorder: Pooled data from two randomized controlled trials. *Aust N Z J Psychiatry.* 2021;55(8):784–798.

STUDY TYPE: Post-hoc analysis of data from two randomized controlled trials

Recent data suggest inflammation may play a role in depression, prompting research into the efficacy of minocycline (a tetracycline antibiotic with anti-inflammatory effects) as an augmenting agent for major depressive disorder (MDD).

Researchers conducted a pooled data analysis from two multisite, double-blinded, placebo-controlled trials of minocycline 200 mg/day taken over 12 weeks. Participants were healthy adults with a diagnosis of non-treatment-resistant, moderate to severe MDD already receiving treatment for depression for the prior two to six weeks. Treatments included antidepressants (86%–89%), antipsychotics (29%–30%), and benzodiazepines (36%–40%).

RESULTS:

Patients (n=112) who were randomized to adjunctive minocycline (n=57) were twice as likely as those on placebo (n=55) to show a response to treatment, defined as a greater than 50% reduction in the Hamilton Rating Scale for Depression (HAMD) score. They were also twice as likely to experience remission, defined as a HAMD score less than 7. Specifically, 57% of the minocycline group showed a response to treatment and 32% achieved remission, in comparison to the placebo group, where 23% responded to treatment and 11% experienced remission.

Rates of adverse effects were comparable in the minocycline and placebo groups. Interestingly, the best responders were participants who used pain medications, had a longer duration of illness, and were older.

CARLAT TAKE:
Minocycline is affordable, readily available, and has a low likelihood of producing antibiotic resistance (Husain MI et al, *J Psychopharmacol* 2017;31(9):1166–1175).

PRACTICE IMPLICATIONS:
Consider adding minocycline to your list of augmentation strategies for the treatment of major depression, particularly for patients with pain or longer duration of illness. Be cautious when prescribing to women of reproductive age: Minocycline reduces the efficacy of hormonal contraceptives and should not be used in pregnancy.

How Essential Is Antidepressant Continuation?

REVIEW OF: Lewis G, Marston L, Duffy L, et al. Maintenance or discontinuation of antidepressants in primary care. *N Engl J Med.* 2021;385(14):1257–1267.

STUDY TYPE: Randomized controlled trial

Most of us have been taught that long-term antidepressant therapy is crucial for patients who have had three or more episodes of depression. This idea is based on trials in which patients in remission were randomly assigned to medication continuation versus placebo. Those switched to placebo had a higher rate of relapse, especially if they'd had three prior episodes of depression.

However, these studies had a number of flaws that may bias the results. Generally, patients were in remission for a relatively short time—typically from three to eight months. Second, antidepressant discontinuation was typically done rapidly, making it hard to tell whether patients actually relapsed or were suffering from antidepressant withdrawal symptoms. Third, the switch to placebo took place at a fixed time instead of when patients felt ready to come off their antidepressant. That leaves open the question: Can patients who have been in sustained remission from depression and feel ready to come off medication safely discontinue antidepressants?

In this study, researchers recruited 478 adult patients from 150 general practices across England. All patients had a history of at least two prior depressive episodes, were currently in remission, had been taking their antidepressant for at least nine months, and felt well enough to consider stopping their medication. Only antidepressants that are commonly prescribed and known to have low rates of withdrawal were included: citalopram, sertraline, fluoxetine, and mirtazapine. Consenting patients were randomized in a double-blind manner to either remain on their antidepressant or have it slowly replaced with a placebo over two months (fluoxetine was tapered over only one month due to its long half-life). Patients were then followed every three months for one year to ascertain relapse rates.

RESULTS:

In total, 92 of 238 patients (39%) in the maintenance group relapsed compared to 135 of 240 (56%) in the discontinuation group over the course of 52 weeks (hazard ratio 2.06; $p<0.0001$). Differences in rates of depression, anxiety, and quality of life all emerged within 12 weeks and persisted throughout the trial. Of the patients who stopped their trial medication, 20% of the maintenance group and 39% of the discontinuation group elected to resume antidepressant medication.

One potential limitation of the study was that reported rates of medication withdrawal symptoms were higher in the discontinuation group (3.1) than the maintenance group (1.9; 95% CI [1.5, 2.3]). Although this could represent an unmasking of depressive symptoms, it also suggests that despite the slow taper, physiological withdrawal cannot be ruled out as a contributing factor.

CARLAT TAKE:

This landmark study puts the risks of antidepressant discontinuation in perspective. On the one hand, staying on the medication lowered the relapse risk by 17% over the course of a year. On the other hand, 44% did successfully taper off their antidepressant without relapsing.

PRACTICE IMPLICATIONS:

These results challenge the black-and-white recommendation to remain on an antidepressant indefinitely after more than two episodes of depression and move the question into the realm of collaborative decision-making between clinician and patient.

Lumateperone in Bipolar Depression

REVIEW OF: Calabrese JR, Durgam S, Satlin A, et al. Efficacy and safety of lumateperone for major depressive episodes associated with bipolar I or bipolar II disorder: A Phase 3 randomized placebo-controlled trial. *Am J Psychiatry*. 2021;178(12):1098–1106.

STUDY TYPE: Randomized controlled trial

In 2019, lumateperone (Caplyta) became the 13th atypical antipsychotic with FDA approval for schizophrenia. Compared to other atypicals, it is relatively well tolerated, with low rates of akathisia and metabolic side effects. And as of December 2021, lumateperone now has an indication for depression in bipolar I and II disorders. This study was a Phase 3 trial of lumateperone for bipolar depression.

Researchers conducted a randomized, placebo-controlled, multicenter trial involving 377 patients with both bipolar I (n=301) and II (n=76) depression. The study was "quadruple-blind," meaning the subjects, providers, investigators, and people administering the rating scales were all unaware of the assigned treatment. The primary outcome measure was the clinician-rated Montgomery-Åsberg Depression Rating Scale (MADRS). Lumateperone was started and maintained at 42 mg/day and used as monotherapy.

RESULTS:

After six weeks, lumateperone outperformed placebo with a medium effect size (0.56) on the primary outcome of change on the MADRS. Response (51.1% vs 36.7%; $p<0.001$) and remission rates (39.9% vs 33.5%; $p<0.018$) were also significantly greater with lumateperone. It was well tolerated, with minimal risk of metabolic side effects, extrapyramidal side effects, or hyperprolactinemia. A post-hoc analysis found greater benefits in bipolar II vs bipolar I depression (effect size of 0.81 vs 0.49) and revealed that a subgroup of patients with mixed features benefited from the medication.

In approving lumateperone for bipolar I and II depression, the FDA also reviewed two similar trials. These have not been published but were made available as a press release. One study was negative (Study 401) and the other positive (Study 402). Both were large, six-week trials, enrolling 554 and 529 patients. Unlike the study above, they tested three arms: lumateperone 28 mg, lumateperone 42 mg, and placebo. The positive study tested lumateperone as an adjunct to lithium or valproate; it arrived at a small effect size (0.27) for the 42 mg dose and a nonsignificant effect for the 28 mg dose. These trials were unique in their inclusion of bipolar II patients. Previously, only quetiapine and cariprazine were tested in this population, and only the quetiapine studies were positive.

CARLAT TAKE:

Lumateperone joins quetiapine as the only atypical antipsychotic with evidence in both bipolar I and bipolar II depression.

PRACTICE IMPLICATIONS:
Among the options for bipolar depression, lumateperone stands out for its greater tolerability and demonstrated benefits in bipolar II. Its efficacy, however, is about average for this class, and its effects in mania and hypomania are unknown.

Optimal Antidepressant Doses in Major Depression

REVIEW OF: Furukawa TA, Cipriani A, Cowen PJ, Leucht S, Egger M, Salanti G. Optimal dose of selective serotonin reuptake inhibitors, venlafaxine, and mirtazapine in major depression: A systematic review and dose-response meta-analysis. *Lancet Psychiatry*. 2019;6(7):601–609.

STUDY TYPE: Systemic review and meta-analysis

Most antidepressants do not have a linear response curve. In other words, the benefits level off as the dose goes up. If the dose goes too high, side effects are likely to outweigh those diminishing returns. What's not clear is where the "sweet spot" lies for each antidepressant; this study set out to find that optimal dose range.

This dose-response meta-analysis included 77 double-blind, randomized, placebo-controlled trials of fixed-dose SSRIs (except fluvoxamine), venlafaxine, and mirtazapine in major depression (n=19,365). Trial length was four to 12 weeks, with a median range of eight weeks. Primary outcomes were efficacy (treatment response defined as 50% or greater reduction in depressive symptoms), tolerability (dropouts due to adverse effects), and acceptability (dropouts for any reason).

RESULTS:

The best balance of efficacy, tolerability, and acceptability was achieved with low to medium doses (see table on next page). At higher doses (greater than 40 mg of fluoxetine equivalents), the benefits plateaued, and dropouts from side effects showed steep linear or exponential curves. Venlafaxine was unique in that efficacy did continue to increase up to 375 mg, though slowed at doses above 150 mg.

CARLAT TAKE:
When a patient does not recover fully on an antidepressant, it's tempting to keep raising the dose. That strategy may work in some patients, but this study suggests that for the average patient, it's more likely to cause side effects than therapeutic gains.

PRACTICE IMPLICATIONS:
High-dose antidepressants are best reserved for the roughly 10% of your patients who are—by definition—off the bell curve. If you do go higher, follow the outcome with a rating scale like the Patient Health Questionnaire (PHQ-9) and consider dropping it back down if there isn't clear improvement.

TABLE: Optimal Doses for Major Depressive Disorder

Antidepressant	Optimal Daily Dose
Citalopram	20–40 mg
Escitalopram	10–15 mg
Fluoxetine	20–40 mg
Mirtazapine	15–30 mg
Paroxetine	20–30 mg
Sertraline	50–100 mg
Venlafaxine	75–150 mg

Oral Zuranolone for Postpartum Depression

REVIEW OF: Deligiannidis KM, Meltzer-Brody S, Gunduz-Bruce H, et al. Effect of zuranolone vs placebo in postpartum depression: A randomized clinical trial. *JAMA Psychiatry.* 2021;78(9):951–959. [Published corrections appear in *JAMA Psychiatry* 2022;79(7):740 and *JAMA Psychiatry* 2023;80(2):191]

STUDY TYPE: Randomized controlled trial

Postpartum depression (PPD) is defined in the DSM-5 as any major depressive episode that begins during pregnancy or within four weeks after giving birth. Traditional antidepressants have long been used during this period, but only small studies supporting their efficacy exist, and none have received FDA approval. Brexanolone (Zulresso) is a neuroactive steroid that was approved by the FDA for PPD in 2019. However, this steroid requires 60 hours of continuous intravenous infusion as well as around-the-clock monitoring due to concerns for potential serious adverse effects, such as loss of consciousness.

Zuranolone is an investigational medicine that is structurally similar to brexanolone but can be given orally once a day. Both drugs work on the GABAergic system in a way that is distinct from benzodiazepines, and both are structural analogues of endogenous allopregnanolone.

This was a Phase 3 study testing the safety and efficacy of zuranolone for PPD. 151 women who developed new-onset depression either during their third trimester of pregnancy or within four weeks following birth were enrolled. Patients were randomized to receive either zuranolone 30 mg or placebo over the course of two weeks. The primary outcome measure was improvement on the Hamilton Depression Rating Scale (HAMD-17), and assessments were made on days three, six, nine, 15, and 45.

RESULTS:

On day 15, which was the primary date of interest, depression scores were significantly lower in the zuranolone cohort (-17.8 points) compared to placebo (-13.6 points) (p=0.003; effect size 0.53). Statistically significant effects were apparent as early as day three and were maintained through day 45, which was a full four weeks after treatment had been completed. Significant improvements were also seen in anxiety and global functioning, as well as maternal functioning. Zuranolone was well tolerated, with the most common side effects being somnolence (15%), headaches (9%), and dizziness (8%), although none of these rates differed much from placebo.

CARLAT TAKE:
Zuranolone appears to be a safe and effective option for PPD. Encouragingly, its benefits appear to occur rapidly, and a two-week course of treatment may be all that is needed for significant results.

PRACTICE IMPLICATIONS:
The FDA is reviewing zuranolone for PPD in 2023. If it comes to market, it will offer a much more pragmatic option than brexanolone. However, several questions remain unanswered, such as its safety in breastfeeding and whether its benefits continue beyond the four-week follow-up in this trial.

Quetiapine in Bipolar With OCD

REVIEW OF: Sahraian A, Ghahremanpouri B, Mowla A. Is quetiapine effective for obsessive and compulsive symptoms in patients with bipolar disorder? A randomized, double-blind, placebo-controlled clinical trial. *CNS Spectr.* 2022;27(5):634–638.

STUDY TYPE: Randomized controlled trial

SSRIs are first-line medications for OCD, but they may pose risks of mania and rapid cycling when patients also have bipolar disorder. These two conditions overlap more often than we'd expect by chance, but only one controlled trial has looked at how to treat OCD in bipolar disorder (it was positive and involved topiramate). This eight-week study tested quetiapine for obsessive-compulsive symptoms in patients with stable bipolar disorder.

The patients were adults with bipolar I disorder who were not in an active mood episode but who had active symptoms of OCD. All were on lithium and clonazepam and no other psychotropics. Although the authors did not make a formal diagnosis of OCD, the participants scored in the moderate to severe range (≥17) on the Yale-Brown Obsessive-Compulsive Scale (Y-BOCS).

A total of 47 patients entered the study after other psychiatric, substance use, and medical diseases were excluded. A total of 40 individuals completed the trial, of which half received placebo and half quetiapine. Doses were increased until the patient either became symptom-free or couldn't tolerate more. Patients completed standard clinician-rated scales for OCD (Y-BOCS, the primary outcome), mania (Young Mania Rating Scale [YMRS]), and depression (Hamilton Depression Rating Scale [HAMD]) at weeks zero, four, and eight.

RESULTS:

On average, Y-BOCS scores fell by 9.1 in the quetiapine group and 0.3 in the placebo group. Half of the quetiapine group had a significant response (>34% decrease in Y-BOCS), compared with 5% of the placebo group. The average dose of quetiapine was 325 mg, although the dose range wasn't reported. All patients remained euthymic during the eight-week trial, based on YMRS and HAMD scores.

Of the 47 participants who entered the study, seven dropped out, none for reasons associated with quetiapine. Those who took quetiapine were 2.3 times more likely to report side effects, particularly drowsiness, increased appetite, constipation, and orthostasis.

CARLAT TAKE:

Quetiapine is difficult to tolerate, but it may be worth trying when OCD is causing significant impairment in patients with bipolar disorder. It made a meaningful difference in this study, bringing the Y-BOCS score from the moderate-severe to the mild range.

PRACTICE IMPLICATIONS:

Quetiapine joins topiramate as a "mood-sparing" treatment for those who suffer from both bipolar disorder and OCD symptoms.

Psilocybin: The New Holy Grail for the Rapid Relief of Major Depression?

REVIEW OF: Davis AK, Barrett FS, May DG, et al. Effects of psilocybin-assisted therapy on major depressive disorder: A randomized clinical trial. *JAMA Psychiatry*. 2021;78(5):481–489.

STUDY TYPE: Randomized controlled trial

INTRAVENOUS KETAMINE AND intranasal esketamine (Spravato) offer hope in the search for a rapidly acting antidepressant. However, concerns regarding addiction, safety, and effect durability have prompted searches for alternative rapid-acting treatments. Psilocybin is a hallucinogen found in mushrooms that, like ketamine, is a recreational drug with potential antidepressant effects. This open-label randomized controlled trial (RCT) was the first controlled study to explore its efficacy for depression.

Participants diagnosed with moderate to severe depression, and not taking antidepressants, were randomly assigned to an immediate-treatment group (n=14) or a delayed-treatment/waiting-list control group (n=13). During the initial eight weeks, the immediate-treatment group received three weeks of preparatory therapy followed by two day-long sessions in which they received a lower dose of psilocybin (20 mg/70 kg) in session one and a higher dose (30 mg/70 kg) in session two. During the psilocybin sessions, they received supportive therapy and were encouraged to focus their attention inward as they listened to music. Patients who were randomized to the delayed group were provided this psilocybin protocol after serving as the control for the immediate group. Depression was rated using the GRID-Hamilton Depression Rating Scale (GRID-HAMD).

RESULTS:

The immediate group responded rapidly and significantly compared to the control group. Subjects in the control group experienced no improvement while waiting, but once treated, they responded as robustly as the immediate group on all measures. At one and four weeks after the last drug session, 67% and 71% of pooled treated subjects, respectively, demonstrated a clinically significant response (greater than 50% drop in GRID-HAMD score). At those same one- and four-week measurement points, 58% and 54%, respectively, of treated subjects experienced remission (GRID-HAMD score less than 7).

Psilocybin was well tolerated. The main side effects included vague emotional symptoms (eg, fear, sadness) and physical symptoms (such as a sensation of trembling and mild, transient headaches).

> **CARLAT TAKE:**
> Psilocybin appears to reduce depressive symptoms rapidly and significantly. Additionally, in a follow-up study involving these participants, researchers found response and remission rates of 75% and 58%, respectively, on the GRID-HAMD at 12 months (Gukasyan N et al, *J Psychopharmacol* 2022;36(2):151–158).

PRACTICE IMPLICATIONS:

Psilocybin for depression is promising. With psychedelic research generally, we'll need larger, blinded RCTs, and ideally FDA approval, to use them regularly. When patients come with questions about self-treating, remind them that these studies involve known qualities and quantities of medications in very controlled therapeutic environments. Currently, only experts in jurisdictions where psychedelics are legal should consider recommending them.

The Role of rTMS in Post-Stroke Depression

REVIEW OF: Hordacre B, Comacchio K, Williams L, Hillier S. Repetitive transcranial magnetic stimulation for post-stroke depression: A randomized trial with neurophysiological insight. *J Neurol.* 2021;268(4):1474–1484.

STUDY TYPE: Randomized controlled trial

Post-stroke depression is common, disabling, and often treatment refractory. We know repetitive transcranial magnetic stimulation (rTMS) is effective for treatment-resistant depression. Might it offer a safe and effective treatment for post-stroke depression? Two previous small randomized controlled trials of rTMS demonstrated its safety and efficacy with 1,000 pulses per session for post-stroke depression (Gu SY and Chang MC, *Brain Stimul* 2017;10(2):270–274; Jorge RE et al, *Biol Psychiatry* 2004;55(4):398–405). Researchers in the current study hypothesized that delivery of a higher-dose rTMS protocol of 3,000 pulses at 10 Hz per session would increase clinical benefits without compromising safety.

Eleven patients with moderate post-stroke depression (Patient Health Questionnaire [PHQ-9] score greater than 5) and no change in antidepressant medication for the prior six months were recruited for this study. Most of the patients were male (82%), ages 44–78 years, with predominantly right hemispheric strokes occurring one to 11 years prior to enrollment. Participants were randomized to either active (n=6) or sham (n=5) rTMS groups for 10 sessions over five weekdays for two consecutive weeks. The Beck Depression Inventory-II (BDI) was the primary outcome measure for depression severity. The BDI was assessed at baseline, immediately post-treatment, and at one month follow-up.

RESULTS:

From baseline to one month follow-up, the BDI scores in the treatment group decreased significantly more than in the sham group, with an average change of 12 points ($p=0.04$). Adverse effects were transient and comparable between the treatment and sham groups; they included mild headaches, mild and moderate neck pain, and sleep disturbances.

CARLAT TAKE:
This study was small and only followed moderately depressed patients for one month, but it provides evidence of the efficacy and safety of this rTMS protocol.

PRACTICE IMPLICATIONS:
TMS protocols are being developed and refined for a variety of indications. Higher-dose rTMS of 3,000 pulses per session may be a safe and effective treatment option post-stroke.

PTSD

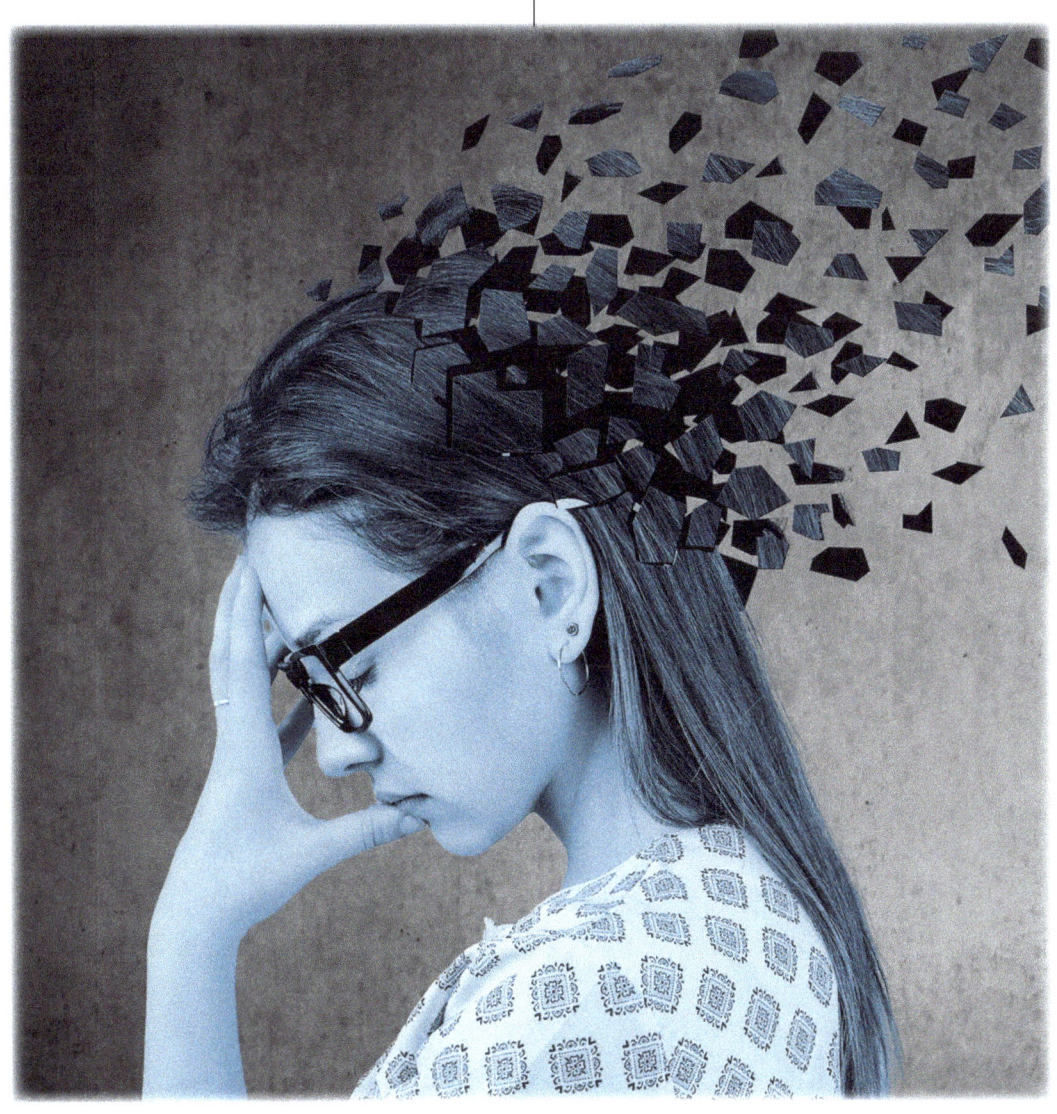

Shining a Light on PTSD

REVIEW OF: Youngstedt SD, Kline CE, Reynolds AM, et al. Bright light treatment of combat-related PTSD: A randomized controlled trial. *Mil Med.* 2022;187(3–4):e435–e444.

STUDY TYPE: Randomized controlled trial

PTSD is difficult to treat, particularly when the trauma is combat related. Numerous interventions for PTSD (eg, prazosin, sertraline, and risperidone) have failed with veterans (Raskind MA et al, *N Engl J Med* 2018;378(6):507–517). This study took a different approach and is the first randomized controlled trial of light therapy for PTSD.

The VA Medical Center in Columbia, South Carolina, randomized 69 veterans with combat-related PTSD (from Afghanistan and/or Iraq) to four weeks of morning bright light treatment or a placebo. Those with a history of winter depression were excluded. Light therapy consisted of 30 minutes of 10,000 lux ultraviolet-filtered white light within one hour of arising. The placebo was an inactivated negative ion generator, which has been used to control for light therapy in other studies. Participants were blindly rated on the Clinician-Administered PTSD Scale (CAPS) and the Clinical Global Impressions Scale (CGI). Self-reported measures of depression, anxiety, side effects, and sleep were elicited at baseline and upon completion of the study. Sleep variables were indirectly measured via continuous wrist actigraphic recording. Approximately two-thirds of the participants in the study were simultaneously receiving other treatments for PTSD. The study was funded by the VA.

RESULTS:

Bright light significantly improved scores on the CAPS and CGI, with a large effect size (1.1) compared to placebo. Additionally, significantly more subjects receiving bright light achieved a response (greater than 33% reduction) compared to placebo (44.1% vs 8.6%). However, no participant achieved remission from PTSD. Remarkably, scores for depression, anxiety, and sleep did not differ between treatment and control. There were no significant side effects with light therapy. Although the subjects were not blinded to their treatment (no pun intended), there was no significant difference in expectation of improvement between treatment and control.

CARLAT TAKE:

Although this is only one study, and subjects weren't blinded, light therapy had a large effect size on symptoms of combat-related PTSD, with few side effects.

Future research comparing light therapy to medications and psychotherapy will further inform our understanding of this modality. Most mental illnesses, including PTSD, are associated with circadian rhythm abnormalities, which may explain some of these benefits. Light therapy also modulates serotonin. However, this doesn't explain why sleep and depression did not improve with light therapy.

PRACTICE IMPLICATIONS:

We don't have many options for combat-related PTSD, and light therapy has a good safety record in depression, although headache and eye strain can occur, and it should be used with caution in ocular disease. Consider it as an augmentation to medications and therapy for PTSD, or for patients who want a non-medication approach or suffer from seasonal depression.

Two Negative Studies of Mirtazapine and Riluzole for PTSD in Veterans

REVIEW OF: Davis LL, Pilkinton P, Lin C, Parker P, Estes S, Bartolucci A. A randomized, placebo-controlled trial of mirtazapine for the treatment of posttraumatic stress disorder in veterans. *J Clin Psychiatry*. 2020;81(6):20m13267.

Spangler PT, West JC, Dempsey CL, et al. Randomized controlled trial of riluzole augmentation for posttraumatic stress disorder: Efficacy of a glutamatergic modulator for antidepressant-resistant symptoms. *J Clin Psychiatry*. 2020;81(6):20m13233.

STUDY TYPE: Two randomized controlled trials

Medications for PTSD don't have a great track record, particularly in combat-related trauma. Prazosin, risperidone, psychotherapy, and the FDA-approved sertraline have all failed in this population. These two trials shed more light on the struggle to find more effective treatments.

Davis' team hypothesized that mirtazapine, with both noradrenergic and serotonergic effects, would improve PTSD by decreasing sleep problems, and perhaps fear and arousal. Mirtazapine has some evidence of efficacy in PTSD, with support from a few controlled but flawed trials (ie, they lacked randomization and placebo). Spangler's team looked at riluzole, a glutamatergic modulator, as an augmenter to an SSRI. Riluzole has open-label data in treatment-resistant depression and anxiety, and is related to glutamatergic agents we already use in psychiatry, like lamotrigine, ketamine, and N-acetylcysteine.

Both studies were done with American veterans with combat-related PTSD, mostly men; only three subjects in the mirtazapine trial had PTSD from other trauma. Other psychiatric and substance diagnoses were excluded from the riluzole trial, but the mirtazapine study allowed comorbid depressive, anxiety, or substance use disorders.

In the riluzole study, 79 subjects already on SSRIs or SNRIs for eight weeks were randomized to receive riluzole (mean dose 126 mg/day) augmentation, or placebo, for eight more weeks. The mirtazapine study randomized 78 subjects to get the active drug (mean dose 39 mg/day) or placebo for eight weeks as monotherapy. The primary outcome measured in both was change in PTSD symptoms as measured by the Clinician-Administered PTSD Scale (CAPS) (for riluzole) or the Structured Interview for PTSD (for mirtazapine). Both studies used standard rating scales to track secondary outcomes for depression, anxiety, sleep, disability, and global function.

RESULTS:

Both drugs failed on the primary PTSD measures. Among secondary measures, riluzole was only positive on the hyperarousal subscale of the CAPS, and mirtazapine only made a significant difference on global functioning. Surprisingly, mirtazapine did not help sleep and appeared to increase nightmares in some subjects. Both medications were well tolerated. Riluzole's main side effects were impaired concentration and fatigue, while mirtazapine tended to cause sedation, nightmares, and irritability.

CARLAT TAKE:
We find no significant flaws with these studies, which found no real benefits of riluzole or mirtazapine for PTSD. It's worth noting that riluzole was tested in a more treatment-resistant population, and both studies were conducted in combat-related PTSD, a group that tends to be less responsive to medication.

PRACTICE IMPLICATIONS:
It's not as gratifying to include negative studies here, but you're not likely to benefit your patients with combat-related PTSD if you prescribe them riluzole or mirtazapine.

About Carlat Publishing

Carlat Publishing was founded by Daniel Carlat, MD. Its flagship publication is *The Carlat Psychiatry Report*. The company also publishes *The Carlat Child Psychiatry Report*, *The Carlat Addiction Treatment Report*, *The Carlat Hospital Psychiatry Report*, and *The Carlat Geriatric Psychiatry Report*. Dr. Carlat is an associate clinical professor of psychiatry at Tufts University. He is also the author of *Drug Metabolism in Psychiatry: A Clinical Guide*, *The Psychiatric Interview*, and *Unhinged*, and co-author of *The Medication Fact Book for Psychiatric Practice*, *Treating Alcohol Use Disorder: A Fact Book*, and *Prescribing Psychotropics: From Drug Interactions to Pharmacogenetics*.

For more information, visit www.thecarlatreport.com.

Contact us at:
info@thecarlatreport.com
866-348-9279

www.ingramcontent.com/pod-product-compliance
Lightning Source LLC
LaVergne TN
LVHW070532070526
838199LV00075B/6759